RAISE YOUR I.Q.

BOOK YOUR PLACE ON OUR WEBSITE AND MAKE THE READING CONNECTION!

We've created a customized website just for our very special readers, where you can get the inside scoop on everything that's going on with Zebra, Pinnacle and Kensington books.

When you come online, you'll have the exciting opportunity to:

- View covers of upcoming books
- Read sample chapters
- Learn about our future publishing schedule (listed by publication month *and author*)
- Find out when your favorite authors will be visiting a city near you
- Search for and order backlist books from our online catalog
- Check out author bios and background information
- Send e-mail to your favorite authors
- Meet the Kensington staff online
- Join us in weekly chats with authors, readers and other guests
- Get writing guidelines
- AND MUCH MORE!

**Visit our website at
http://www.kensingtonbooks.com**

RAISE YOUR I.Q.

STEPHEN LANGER, MD
AND JAMES F. SCHEER

7 ways to boost your mind power—
no matter what your age

Kensington Books
Kensington Publishing Corp.
http://www.kensingtonbooks.com

This publication and product is designed to provide accurate and authoritative information with regard to the subject matter covered. The purchase of this publication does not create a doctor-patient relationship between the purchaser and the author, nor should the information contained in this book be considered specific medical advice with respect to a specific patient and/or specific condition. In the event the purchaser desires to obtain specific medical advice or other information concerning a specific person, condition, or situation, the services of a competent professional should be sought.

The author and publisher specifically disclaim any liability, loss, or risk, personal or otherwise, that is or may be incurred as a consequence, directly or indirectly, of the use and application of any of the information contained in this book.

KENSINGTON BOOKS are published by

Kensington Publishing Corp.
850 Third Avenue
New York, NY 10022

Copyright © 1999 by Stephen Langer, M.D., and James F. Scheer

All rights reserved. No part of this book may be reproduced in any form or by any means without the prior written consent of the Publisher, excepting brief quotes used in reviews.

Kensington and the K logo Reg. U.S. Pat. & TM Off.

First Printing: June, 1999
10 9 8 7 6 5 4 3 2 1

Printed in the United States of America

I dedicate this book to
My wife Debra
My daughter Caroline and
My brother Stuart
   I love you all.
      Stephen E. Langer, M.D.

I dedicate this book to
My wife Joan with thanks and gratitude for her
support and encouragement in writing this book.
                    With all my love,
                         James F. Scheer

Contents

Acknowledgments 9
Introduction 11

1. Making of a Genius 15
2. Exercise the Brain for Better Thinking! 25
3. The Importance of Being Oxygenated 37
4. Nutrients That Skyrocket Your I.Q. 53
5. Brain Transplant or Something Better? 70
6. CATS and Your Mind 79
7. Heavy Metals and Your Brain 94
8. Stress: The Mind-Killer 103
9. How to Boost Your Memory 120
10. The Answers to Alzheimer's Disease? 135
11. Hormones for the Head 148
12. How to Raise Your Child's I.Q.—Part One 164
13. How to Raise Your Child's I.Q.—Part Two 182
14. The Summing Up 205
    Appendix: Exotic Brain Boosters 212

References 223
Recommended Reading 237

Introduction

"Between our birth and death, we may touch understanding as a moth brushes a window with its wings."

These words of wisdom from writer Christopher Fry apply to many of us—if not most of us—relative to knowledge in general and knowledge about the mind's capabilities and potentials in particular.

The purpose of this book is to make you aware of your unrealized, hidden, mental capabilities and potentials, and to show you how to expand and enhance them.

It seems that the currents in the life of health editor and writer James F. "Jim" Scheer, my collaborator, and those in my life moved us almost purposefully to resource individuals and research studies that made us realize a book on this subject was necessary. These currents also made us realize that we were particularly qualified to write it.

Jim was blessed with being closely associated with pioneers and giants in health and nutrition, the following legendary medical doctors: Francis M. Pottenger, Jr., Joseph Risser, W. Coda Martin, W.D. Currier, and Broda O. Barnes—among others. They and biochemist Michael Walsh, Sci.D., made him aware that whole foods, fresh vegetables, fruits, and super-supplements contribute as much to a sound, bright mind, efficient memory, and emotional stability as to a perfectly healthy body.

The profound effect on mind and body of high octane foods and supplements excited Jim when he saw "before" and "after" photos of patients lining all four walls of the large waiting room of Dr. Pottenger's Monrovia, California, offices. Many patients had emerged from life-draining illnesses and, lean and bony, looked as if they had suffered the privations of a concentration camp. In their "after" photos, they could have qualified to appear on the covers of body beautiful magazines.

With super-foods and regular aerobic exercise, many also showed a remarkable rise in I.Q. and improvement in memory, impressing Jim with the fact that feeding the body properly also feeds the mind. In addition, it was Dr. Pottenger who introduced Jim to the work of Dr. Weston Price, a Cleveland doctor of dental surgery.

Dr. Price's studies of primitive cultures throughout the world demonstrated graphically the merits of whole foods for healthy bodies and bright minds. His studies underscored the need for special diets to prepare both wives and husbands for pregnancy to assure having healthy and intelligent infants.

My fascination with upgrading the mind by superbly feeding the body came also from reading Weston Price's book, *Nutrition and Physical Degeneration,* which more generally showed the subtle, yet harmful, effects of processed foods. My own patients brought further proof—remarkable mental improvements through super-nutrition.

Further, patients' probing questions about biochemical enhancement of Intelligence Quotient induced me to search the literature for more answers. I was awed by the positive evidence there and dismayed that so little of it had appeared in popular books.

Introduction 13

This discovery made Jim and me determined to offer a book that covered every aspect of reviving the mind and memory to cope and—more than that—succeed in a highly competitive world.

In these pages, you will discover ways to develop your powers of concentration and memory beyond belief. You will help yourself to greater self-fulfillment and a more abundant life.

You'll discover breakthroughs in super-nutrition, anti-aging hormones, advanced learning, stress reduction, and mental gymnastics. No matter what your sex or age—middle-school to super-seniority—you can benefit beyond expectation.

Many solid studies and my clinical experiences not only show that this can be done, but that it can be done with dramatic and spirit-elevating results. These results will not only change *your* life, but the lives of everyone around you.

There are seven major ways to make your I.Q. skyrocket and your memory cling to vital information. These will be offered in the following pages, along with other ways of related importance.

We thank you for giving us the opportunity to share with you the greatest available stimulants to mind and memory. We wish you the best for good health and prosperity.

Stephen Langer, M.D.
Berkeley, California

CHAPTER 1

Making of a Genius

You can become a genius in the short time it will take you to read this book and apply its simple information!

Impossible!

See for yourself in the pages that follow. For openers, consider results achieved by Professor Robert Rivera. He regularly boosts the Intelligence Quotients (I.Q.s) of students from average—110 to 120—by as much as 30 points into the genius level.[1]

Rivera doesn't do it with mirrors, just with a common-sense system that's yours for the taking. A memory expert and speech teacher at Valley College in Van Nuys, California, Professor Rivera achieves this mind miracle by using sound principles of physiology.

Super-efficient blood flow for special delivery of oxygen and nutrients to the brain are the major rocket boosters for the I.Q. Almost any aerobic exercise done for 15 or 20 minutes will rev up your ability to think and remember more efficiently.

Professor Rivera, however, accomplishes more and does it even easier and in less time with two simple physical exercises that produce phenomenal results. His students who use them before quizzes and final exams routinely get the highest grades.

Coached by Professor Rivera, business executives also use them before critical meetings or prior to writing crucial reports or winning proposals for contracts.

Here's how the Rivera system works.

Inhale for eight counts. Hold your breath for 12 counts, then slowly exhale for 10 counts. Professor Rivera suggests repeating this exercise 10 times. Remember this though: If you start feeling dizzy, stop right away; if there's the least question about the condition of your health, don't do the exercises without the approval of a qualified health professional.

His second exercise requires that you stand and flatten yourself against a wall, then stretch upward. Do this 10 times. Some people practice both routines and experience a major I.Q. blast-off. Rivera also advises sitting up straight at your desk for maximum brain efficiency. A bowed back and rounded shoulders are thought to reduce blood circulation to the brain.

Perform the Rivera routines several times daily, and you'll be at the peak of your thinking ability.

Having studied the thinking habits and practices of respected minds over the years, Professor Rivera recognized the major physiological reason for their success: "It's simple. Geniuses have better blood flow to their brains!"

Brains in Good Standing

Not long ago Dr. Max Vercruyssen, a human factors professor and researcher at the University of Southern California, revealed that standing rather than sitting dramatically enhances the ability to learn and think.[2]

He found this out by studying one hundred adults of

assorted ages who were given computer tasks to perform for 15 minutes while standing and, then, while sitting.

In a news story released by the university, Dr. Vercruyssen announced that "performance ratings ranged from five to 30 percent higher for the subjects while they were standing."

On the basis of this study, he makes the following recommendation: "When at work performing tasks that require mental activity, periodically stand up to help improve your thinking and cognitive ability."

Although authorities in this area are not sure why you think better on your feet, Dr. Vercruyssen theorizes that this might be related to the genetic fight or flight pattern in which a startled individual quickly jumps to his or her feet ready to fight or run. Dr. Vercruyssen feels that both your body and brain are poised for action when you stand.

Assuredly, standing revs up the metabolism more than just sitting. Let me share with you a personal experience. While in medical college, I used to study or memorize as I walked around the room. My roommate thought I was ridiculous. But as the USC study substantiates, I was doing the right thing. I get the same great results today when I read and pace. That's the bottom line.

Couch Potatoes Stunt Their Brains

Although we know that the brain has a profound influence on the body, we sometimes overlook the fact that the body influences the brain, too. We also overlook the fact that the brain is a physical organ that needs some physical exercise.

For example, in a study at Scripps College, California, researchers found that those who exercised routinely outperform couch potatoes in complex thinking, ability to remember more, and reacting faster.[3]

In another study, a team of University of Alabama

researchers led by K.A. Shay divided 105 men into six groups according to age—young, middle-aged and old—and according to physical fitness—high or low. The men were tested on four kinds of thinking related to attention span, words, simple motor tasks, and complex visual problems.[4]

On three of the four tasks—attention, words, and simple motor function—the physically fit and unfit ended up with almost the same achievement level. In complex visual tasks, however, the physically fit group was definitely superior. This discovery is significant in that it's the complex visual area where sharp declines take place as people age. So being physically active seems to fortify the aging mind where it needs it the most.

At a recent meeting of the American Society for the Advancement of Anti-Aging Medicine, Dharma Singh Khalsa, M.D., noted neurologist and author, stressed these four pillars for keeping the brain young: optimal nutrition (including supplements), stress management, anti-aging drugs, and aerobic conditioning.[5] All four factors will be covered in depth in later chapters.

Speaking to a group of media people, he emphasized one of the pillars, stating that "aerobic exercise stimulates the synthesis of the hormone called 'nerve growth factor' needed to repair neurons. Further, it increases blood flow to the brain and aids in the production of norepinephrine, a neurotransmitter used by the brain to carry short-term memories into long-term storage in the neocortex. Physical exercise is also an excellent reducer of stress and producer of endorphins."

Seven Ways to a Brighter Brain

As important as physical exercises are to super-charging the brain, there are at least six additional ways to upgrade mental abilities: (1) practicing simple thinking exercises; (2) improving nutrition including natural foods; (3) adding low-cost super-supplements to enrich an excellent diet; (4) ridding the brain and body of widespread environmental pollutants; (5) coping with mind-sapping stress, and (6) using natural and safe hormonal brain stimulants.

Let's look at a specific example illustrating each of these categories before exploring them more fully in the chapters to come. Let's also consider information about enhancing memory and keeping the brain young at any age, as well as preventing or coping with mental disease.

Accenting the importance of mental exercise, Professor Rivera also explained that:

> The functional difference between the average brain and that of a genius is an increased flow of blood and oxygen to the brain of the genius through veins and arteries of the meninges (the casings) of the three brain sections. This blood and oxygen flow is improved through mental as well as physical exercise.

A four-year experiment by Dr. John Stirling Meyer and colleagues at Baylor College of Medicine–Houston bears this out.[6]

In this experiment, researchers gave standard neurological and psychological tests to 83 healthy participants averaging 65 years of age and employed at the start of the study, at least. Researchers also took a measure of blood flow to the brain of each participant. Everyone was normal for this age group.

A third of the volunteers kept on working. Another one-third retired but remained active mentally and physically. The remaining one-third retired and became inactive, figuratively storing their brains and bodies in mothballs.

Four years later, the inactive group showed less blood

flow to their brains and, significantly, a far lower I.Q. level than those in the other groups.

Laying it right on the line, Dr. Meyer stated that the declines in blood flow and I.Q. were definitely causally related—the only difference between the groups being their level of mental and physical activity.

Other human as well as animal studies point in the same direction, as our full chapter on this subject will show.

Upgrading the I.Q.

Improved nutrition also frequently produces higher intelligence and problem-solving ability. In my preventive medical practice, I never stop being amazed at this relationship. Almost invariably, patients in ill-health who go on my special regimen regain their health and report better concentration and memory.

The regimen I recommend is to minimize or eliminate junk food and to consume a diet rich in whole grain cereals and breads made from them, seeds and nuts, and fresh enzyme-rich fruits and vegetables. I also recommend that my patients begin each day with a high protein breakfast to help super-charge their mental and physical energy until noon. Then I request of all my patients that they take a supplemental multivitamin, as well as calcium-magnesium, and vitamin C.

One patient in particular comes to mind here: a young woman, a junior at the nearby University of California at Berkeley. Early this year, she took an I.Q. test and scored 118. Four months later, after staying on my regimen religiously, she was tested again. This time she was elated about her score of 130.

"I came to you because I was always so tired I could hardly drag myself to classes. Now I feel great physically and—the unexpected reward—I tested higher than ever before on my I.Q. test."

A whole chapter on the subject of brain nutrients could be written, and it will be—later in this book.

Super-supplements added to a largely natural food diet can make dramatic differences in mental ability and achievement.

Remarkable Results

The unexpected mental results from upgraded diets has made me a student of every report I can get my hands on. Nutrient supplementation for better thinking and memory is now an important part of my preventive medical practice.

Another patient—let's call her Renee—a young woman who was nervous about a crucial, after-work interview for a better job, was almost in tears during her appointment in my offices.

"After a super-stressed workday, I'm brain dead," she confessed. "What can I do?"

Thanks to the extensive research by Drs. Richard J. Wurtman and Judith Wurtman at Massachusetts Institute of Technology, I recommended that, before her interview, she eat a light dinner with foods rich in the amino acid tyrosine, to spark her thinking and raise her blood sugar level.

The best bets for tyrosine-rich foods are cottage cheese (my patient was not milk-intolerant or milk-allergic), turkey, duck, tuna fish, tofu, and wheat germ. Tyrosine is important because it helps produce the key brain stimulants norepinephrine and dopamine.

I'm pleased to say that she followed my recommendations, had a brilliant interview, and won the new position and a substantially higher salary. She later told me, "I've never felt brighter or more lucid in my thinking and talking."

The very same formula worked for a friend before his

CPA exam and for a trial lawyer patient before the climax of the biggest case of her life.

Over and above meals containing tyrosine, I suggest that patients take supplements that stimulate their brain and recharge a delinquent and undependable memory. Key brain supplements include ginkgo biloba, which increases blood flow throughout the body, particularly the brain; glutamine and cysteine (necessary for the body to synthesize glutathione), an efficient free radical killer; phenylalanine, which raises blood levels of the brain-stimulating neurotransmitter norepinephrine; pyroglutamic acid; acetyl-L-carnitine; choline; and vitamin B complex. Glutathione and superoxide dismutase (SOD) are inner guards that protect delicate nerve cells of the brain from attack by free radicals, unstable and damaging molecules. All these factors will be discussed in detail later.

Toxins Dull the Mind

Taking super-supplements to stimulate the brain yet may not be enough. You must also protect your body-mind from environmental toxins that can slow your ability to think clearly and quickly.

Among the most hazardous mind-robbing pollutants are lead, cadmium, mercury, and carbon monoxide from the exhaust pipes of cars and trucks. Perhaps the most notorious of these is lead.

When we compare the level of lead found in people today with levels found in skeletons of individuals who lived in the 1500s, we learn the shocking fact that we carry a lead load 500 percent greater than they. Lead is present in food, water, and air, even though leaded gasoline has been banned in the United States for many years.

Numerous studies show that lead causes a multitude of neurological problems, reduces I.Q., causes memory loss, and makes it difficult for some individuals to maintain balance and motor control.

We know that pregnant women and children are most susceptible to brain problems due to lead. In the womb and in the earliest years when the brain is developing most rapidly, lead pollution can cause the most serious damage—sometimes irreversible.

Still other studies disclose that children living in the heart of industrial cities, where lead levels are highest, score eight to ten percent lower in I.Q. measurements than those in lower lead areas such as the suburbs.

No one is safe from lead. There are, however, many ways to limit our intake of this pollutant and to rid ourselves of the lead already deposited in our brains and body cells. These will be elaborated in the full chapter on brain-sabotaging pollutants.

And how many of us are aware of how stress can reduce—in some cases, even undermine—our thinking and memory?

How Brain Cells Get Injured

A study at the Salk Institute in La Jolla, California, shows that stress can severely harm brain function, because it diverts the brain's favorite food, glucose, to other vital organs and to muscle systems in response to the stress emergency.[7]

This glucose deprivation injures cells in the hippocampus, a brain area devoted to memory and mood control. Sustained stress is particularly damaging because glucose deprivation can bring on brain cell starvation and, in extreme cases, even death.

Sadly, certain forms of stress are so subtle that many people are not aware of them and, thus, cannot avoid or alleviate them. The complete chapter on stress and reduced thinking and memory will also disclose how to detect subtle stressors and eliminate them.

The brain can also be sabotaged by too little natural hormones—thyroid, DHEA, melatonin, and human growth hormone. For example, an estimated 40 percent of adults in the United States may be suffering—many unknowingly—from clinical or subclinical low thyroid functioning (hypothyroidism).

Most sophisticated tests for thyroid are specific for this disease but often inaccurate, missing many subtle cases of hypothyroidism, which may cause up to 64 symptoms, among them: cold hands and feet, overwhelming fatigue, sexual inadequacy, female problems and—most pertinent to this book—sluggish thinking and faulty memory.

Unfortunately, many of the brain symptoms of hypothyroidism are mistaken for senile dementia or Alzheimer's disease. Once detected though, they are easily correctible, either with applied clinical nutrition or with Armour natural thyroid, a prescription drug.

A Free Medical Test?

There's a simple, no-cost test that you can use to determine whether or not you are hypothyroid. It's called the Barnes Basal Temperature Test, which we will describe how to perform in Chapter 3 on maximizing brain function with thyroid supplementation.[8] Further, we will show how to compensate for too little natural hormone with the synthetic hormones DHEA, melatonin, pregnenolone, and human growth hormone to develop a sky-high I.Q. and a razor sharp memory!

Join us in the chapters that follow. You will be doing a favor to yourself, your mind, and your memory!

CHAPTER 2

Exercise the Brain for Better Thinking!

Before going deeply into how to make the brain more physically and mentally fit, let's spend a page or two on what the brain is and how it works.

That brain of yours is a mass of gelatinous cells—as many as 100 billion to 100 trillion cells, depending upon who's keeping score. Those cells make it possible for you to think and remember through communications channels so complicated that you may find it hard to believe that they came about by evolution alone.

Although your brain accounts for just two percent of your body weight, it uses more than 20 percent of your oxygen. Its major food is glucose, a form of sugar. Combined with oxygen and thyroid hormone, your brain burns up about a teaspoon of glucose every hour.

A myth worth shattering is that you use only a fraction of the normal amount of oxygen when you sleep. No way! You use about 97 percent of normal, write the experts.

Your brain receives and transmits messages through networks of neurons (nerves). Too tiny to be seen with the naked eye, each neuron is made up of three parts: dendrites, cell body, and axon.

Dendrites, shaped like tree branches, receive messages transmitted through neurotransmitters, mini chemical tears. The cell's body is like the control tower at an airport. It receives the signal and decides how to act upon it so fast that it makes lightning seem slow in comparison. Next it speeds the message to the axon, a tiny pencil-like shaft that releases the proper neurotransmitter to carry out the order.

There are more than 50 neurotransmitters. The most famiiar are acetylcholine, serotonin, and norepinephrine. Every time someone establishes that there is a certain number of neurotransmitters, a researcher comes up with a new one!

The best known neurotransmitters carry out orders that promote anger, anxiety, alertness, hunger, thirst, sexual appetite, sleepiness or memory. Cell receptors are highly specialized, so that they can accept neurotransmitters of only a certain chemical formula. Like every other part of the body, neurons must be fed properly in order to have a rich supply of neurotransmitters to release when appropriate. An undersupply of the right nutrients can disrupt the harmony of the entire concert of neurotransmitters and contribute to marginal or poor thinking or remembering.

Let's just use a few neurotransmitters as examples. Acetylcholine is made from choline, supplied mainly by soybeans, liver, and eggs or by a nutritional supplement such as lecithin, phosphatidylcholine, or choline itself.

Tryptophan, an amino acid found in turkey, chicken, and milk, is the forerunner of the neurotransmitter serotonin. Unfortunately, tryptophan is not readily absorbed. When ingested with other amino acids, it doesn't muscle its way to get a seat on the train. Other more aggressive amino acids crowd it out. To eliminate the competition, it is best to take tryptophan along with some carbohydrate and vitamin B–6. If your body is running low on niacin, it can convert tryptophan into this vitamin.

Tyrosine, found in most foods, is transformed by your body into the neurotransmitter epinephrine.

Let's let neurologist Jay Lombard and Carl Germano explain succinctly and colorfully how communication takes place here:

> Neurotransmitters are the brain's pony express messengers, chemicals that leap across tiny gaps, or synapses, between brain cells.... Each of your neurons has certain receptors—(there are as many as 100,000 in some instances)—on their cell surfaces, which we call membranes, and these receptors act as receiving platforms for messages from various neurotransmitters.
>
> This exacting process requires a specific match between the receptor and the neurotransmitter, much as every lock requires a specific key. Once a specific neurotransmitter binds to a neuron receptor, it sets a chain reaction into motion within the cell. These chemical reactions in turn regulate and control every cellular process, producing specific biological effects.

The major neurotransmitters are acetylcholine, dopamine, gamma-aminobutyric acid (GABA), glutamate, nitric oxide, norepinephrine, and serotonin. They all have a specific assortment of uses.

Acetylcholine is concerned mainly with thinking, memory, motor coordination, and sleep. An acute lack of it is usually related to Alzheimer's disease.

Dopamine is important to the control of movement and to the function of the brain. A dopamine deficiency is said to contribute to the tremors and involuntary movements of Parkinson's disease.

GABA serves as a biochemical brake to keep nerves from firing too fast so that brain systems don't become overloaded and destroy healthy neurons. It usually balances glutamate, an energy-supplier that sometimes does the over-exciting. However, too little calming from GABA can sometimes result in anxiety or even epileptic seizures.

Nitric oxide, only recently investigated by researchers, helps to govern, maintain, and mend the connection between the brain and the immune system. It also is involved in memory.

Norepinephrine stimulates you in the face of stress. Sometimes it overstimulates. It speeds up your heart rate and breathing. Insufficient norepinephrine can lead to overfatigue, depression, and anxiety.

Serotonin is important to sleeping, appetite, sexual behavior, and to lowering the intensity of pain. A deficiency may cause depression, obsessive-compulsive behavior, eating disorders, inability to sleep, and exaggeration of pain in general.

This background information relates to why your brain thinks and remembers better when it is given regular mental workouts, just as the body functions better due to regular physical exercise. Mental exercise is not a new idea, although an excellent one.

A generation ago, Professor Edward L. Bennett, of the University of California's Laboratory of Biodynamics, headed a research project that pointed today's researchers in this direction.[2]

In an experiment with rats—the four-legged variety—he and associates divided very young animals from the same litter into two groups. They kept one group in bare cages with no prompts or challenges to learning. They gave the other group toys and apparatus that caused them to make complex movements and to solve problems.

Thirty days later, they compared the unchallenged and the challenged rats according to the size of significant parts of the brain and chemical substances in them. The blood vessels of the challenged rats were much wider than those of unchallenged animals, permitting a greater blood flow.

Their brains increased in size. Those of the unchallenged didn't.

Dr. Bennett was quoted as follows: "What we have discovered suggests that training, education, adventure, sports, and other 'experiences' change the brain's chemical and mechanical power for the better."

Exercising the brain makes the brain bigger, just as muscle exercise makes the muscle bigger and more efficient. Asked if he thought results indicate that youthful brains could be retained for longer, Dr. Bennett said that this possibility seems likely.

A generation later, Professor Marian Diamond, a neurobiologist at the University of California, continues this work and produces even more convincing evidence that brain exercises do make the brain larger and more able to solve problems.[3]

Despite such evidence, many of us still think that the brainpower we have today is all we'll ever have, so this limiting attitude defuses our blast-off to a sky-high I.Q.

Thanks to a generation worth of experience seeing successions of rats raise their I.Q.s appreciably, Dr. Diamond has taken the cue. She advises us to optimize ourselves, to seek change, challenge, new experiences, and "never to retire from learning."

Making the "Impossible" Possible

If we seek challenge and constant stimulation in our thinking, we can delay or even defeat mental aging and even develop new brain cells. Only a handful of years ago, this was thought to be impossible.

And the "impossible" is even possible for oldsters among us, because Dr. Diamond discovered that there can be brain growth even in rats who are 80 to 90 years old in human years.

She proved this by moving rats who had lived boring lives in uninteresting cages, with only a few companions into what she calls "enriched living quarters," larger cages with many toys and often 12 other rat companions, where the toys—that is, the challenges—were changed daily.

What sorts of toys? Jungle gyms, little ladders, mazes, swings, treadmills, wheels, balls, and other stimulating items that the rats looked forward to climbing on or pushing around.

Dr. Diamond compared the mental progress of these rats with the progress of those in standard, boring cages who had only a few companions. Rats in the enriched environment thrived mentally and physically, socializing and having fun with their new toys. The other rats were bored, deep in the same rut of routine, keeping to themselves, hardly moving and acting old.

When the experiment ended and the rats were more than 120 years old in human terms, those in the enriched environments were found to have increased their number of brain cells. Their cerebral cortex was six percent thicker than that of the bored-to-death rats, and, more amazingly, their brains contained nine percent less aging pigment (lipofuscin).

And there's even more. When examined microscopically, the rat brains, from the stimulated group showed 24 percent more glial cells in their grey matter than in the grey matter of unstimulated animals. Glial cells support and nourish brain cells (neurons).

Does this mean that, like lab animals, we human beings can grow new brain cells? My collaborator, Jim Scheer, directed this question to Arnold Scheibel, Ph.D., professor of neurology at the University of California at Los Angeles.

"Quite a bit of new research indicates that we can grow new cells in two specific areas of the brain: the hippocampal dentate and the olfactory bulb," said Dr. Scheibel. "The first area is quite important in that our short-term memory storage is in the hippocampus."

For her part, Dr. Diamond conjectured that active healthy brains develop more glial cells per neuron than inactive brains. In her lab, she already had glial cell data from studies of 11 brains of men from ages 49 to 80 to support her conjecture.

The Secret of Einstein's Brain

Then came the most exciting information of her life. Preserved in alcohol and stored in a cardboard box in Kansas was the brain of Albert Einstein, certainly one of the great thinkers of the century. It was possessed by Thomas Harvey, M.D., the pathologist who had performed the autopsy on Einstein, who had died at 76 in a Princeton, New Jersey, hospital. Before dying, Einstein had authorized his brain's removal for research, entrusted to Dr. Harvey.

Oh, to compare—or contrast—the Einstein brain with data from the 11 men already studied! Explaining her research interest—no, fascination—Dr. Diamond wrote to Dr. Harvey, requesting that he send her Einstein brain samples.

Nothing happened for three years, and then, unexpectedly, a brown paper wrapped package arrived at her campus office. It contained plastic capsules with four "superbly preserved" three-quarter-inch-cube samples of Albert Einstein's brain from the right and frontal lobes and the right and left lower parietal lobes—areas for abstract thinking.

Dr. Diamond and associates cut slices 6 one-thousandth of a millimeter thick, stained them with a dye so that they could differentiate glial cells from neurons and put them on slides of microscopes. Then they counted both types of cells and compared them with counts for the other 11 brains.

The ratio of glial cells to neurons in Einstein's brain was higher on average than that of the 11, but the difference was small in three samples. In the fourth sample—that from the left parietal lobe, involved in higher math and language abilities—the difference was amazing. Einstein's brain had a ratio of glial cells 73 percent greater than in the other brains.

"The particular area of the brain we examined is responsible for associative thinking, linking ideas together," Dr. Diamond told the press. "So you might say that Einstein was gifted not only in making associations, but also at making associations between associations."

Dr. Diamond then explained her findings with the rats. Challenged brain cells show an expansion of dendrites, the tree-like branches. Additional stimulation often creates more out-branchings.

Where dendrite out-branchings take place, glial cells increase to give physical and nutritional support to nerve cells that do the thinking and reasoning. So challenges and an alive mind apparently cause dendrite growth and expansion and an interrelating of billions of other dendrites, forming a greater internet of communication.

Stimulated Brains Can Grow!

Skeptics may still want more proof than Dr. Diamond has given us, and especially as her findings apply to *human beings*. The proof is all around us, she responds. Stimulated people stay more mentally acute and active and, therefore, younger for longer. Besides, she adds, as brains are essentially large clumps of nerve cells, and nerve cells of rats and human beings contain the same basic constituents, comparisons here are instructive.

She continues: Nerve cells were created to receive stimuli and will react to stimuli at any age. Brains that meet challenges positively don't lose cells; they gain them. We can rev up our I.Q.s and keep them revved up for longer—possibly even a lifetime—by learning, by getting a higher education from this valuable animal research.

Human resarch performed by Maria G. Boorsalis and

Exercise the Brain for Better Thinking! 33

David Snowdon, Ph.D., professor of preventive medicine at the Sanders-Brown Center on Aging at the University of Kentucky, bears out the findings of Dr. Diamond.[4]

Snowdon's continuing study of the aged nuns of the School Sisters of Notre Dame in Mankato, Minnesota, has been publicized in newspapers, magazines, on radio and TV, and yet it is surprising how few people know about them.

Dr. Snowdon discovered that nuns who stay mentally and physically active in challenging activity live longer and their minds and memory stay sharper than those of others and, for the most part, fend off senile dementia and Alzheimer's disease.

Nuns who continue to take college courses, who teach, and who eagerly stay attuned to current events around the world—those constantly challenged—live longer and stay mentally sound longer than the less educated and challenged nuns devoted to cleaning rooms, shopping, and working in the kitchen.

Beware of Routines

We now know that both parts of brain nerves—dendrites and axons—wither with age and disuse. We also know that continued problem-solving expands the tree-like dendrites to create new connections and new networks of nerve connections.

But beware of routine! Once new abilities and skills become routine, the axons and dendrites may shrink. New mental challenges renew them and stimulate regrowth—a good reason for the elderly, especially those with habitual routines, to break out, renew, and regrow these vital brain components.

And what about supplies in reserve? Snowdon and other leading neurologists feel that unceasing mental challenge leads to such a buildup of dendrites and axons that there is a reserve for emergencies. For example, if the neural circuitry in the brain develops the "tangles" characteristic of Alzheimer's disease—as in memory loss—there is still enough circuitry left for messages to be rerouted.

In fact, the abundant neuronal circuitry in the brain is also helpful to the 500,000 Americans who suffer strokes each year. We know this because we can see it. Even a stroke can't keep a good brain down!

Let's return to the nuns now. Aside from staying abreast of news, forming opinions and discussing them—sometimes debates occur—the School Sisters of Notre Dame watch TV quiz shows and often have the right answers before show participants. At the present writing, five of the nuns are more than 100 years old, and their brains are as alive as those of the brightest college students.

Lower Rate of Alzheimer's Disease

Snowdon and associates secured permission from the nuns to conduct autopsies and examine and analyze their brains for the sake of medicine and science. The surviving nuns were eager to learn more about brains and longevity from them.

Looking for signs of senile dementia and Alzheimer's disease, the Snowdon team found an indication of Alzheimer's disease in about 40 percent of the sisters in the group 85 years or older. This compares with 50 percent from the general population.

Dr. Snowdon and most other researchers in this field demonstrate that challenge and activity can preserve sound minds. Stephen Ceci, professor of human development and family studies at Cornell University, gathered results of 200 diverse research projects worldwide over several decades.

His conclusion? That time spent in school has a great influence on a person's I.Q.—more than the quality of the education itself. Assignments and interactions are constant challenges. A strong correlation exists between grade level completed and in I.Q. scores, he finds.[5]

Along a similar line, a 30-year-long study by Dr. K. Warner Schaie, accents the importance of mental stimulation and blasts the notion that we have no control over declining mental abilities.[6]

Dr. Schaie found that people who lead active lives with new experiences showed no significant drop-off of mental acuity after age 60. People who live dull and unstimulating lives showed a marked decline in mental acuity.

Schaie advises people to work crossword puzzles, compete with TV quiz show contestants from the couch, play word games, and learn to square dance—the latter not only for its mental challenge, but also for its fine aerobic exercise.

This Is Your Right Time

The best time in life to accept challenge and stimulation? Anytime. But the earlier you do so, the better you'll be for it! Isolation can slow thinking and remembering. We are in charge of our present. We can reject becoming self-imposed hermits. We can socialize. We can meet challenging people and challenging ideas in newspapers, magazines or books—on the Internet, on TV or on radio. We can limber up our brains by exercises, by thinking up solutions to problems such as widespread use of narcotics, how to provide shelter for the homeless, how to make Social Security more secure, and so on.

We may not come up with the right answers, but we can keep our brains active and young. Some of my patients exercise their minds by trying to remember the definitions of little-used words, by thinking of solutions for their own problems or those of relatives and friends. Some plan a home business—particularly figuring out how to start with little or no money.

Others exercise their minds by reading titles of fiction books, motion pictures, or plays and figuring out their plots. Now that creative exercise is mental aerobics! Then they read the books, see the movies or plays to learn how they came out. What does it matter if their plot is different? It's the mental exercise that counts.

Unsuspected Talent Rewarded

One of my middle-aged patients became so good at that game that she suddenly realized she had unsuspected creative abilities, and so she's doing what she had never done before: writing short stories. She sold one recently. Now nothing can stop her new career. You think that imagining can't help you stay young and active? Think again!

You have a choice. It's never too early or too late to make it. You can stay young all your life and enjoy it to the hilt, or you can isolate yourself from people and stimulating experiences, stop using your mind and start losing it, watch yourself deteriorate and age rapidly. It's really up to you.

Some years ago the Russians conducted a special study of the mental and physical abilities of 21,000 elderly individuals. As presented at the United Nations, the Russian scientists found what we found: "The more that brains and muscles are used, the better they are, and the less they age."

CHAPTER 3

The Importance of Being Oxygenated

A certain simple fact of life sometimes escapes our attention: Being stimulated mentally means being stimulated physically.

As a result, blood flows faster to our trillions of brain and body cells. The rate at which oxygen and food combine to create energy (metabolism) speeds up.

This energy comes from "burning" glucose, the brain's major fuel. Your car's engine needs fuel and oxygen to run. So do *you*. With limited oxygen, the burning of fuel slows down and, along with it, our physical and mental processes. In effect, you can't think and remember as efficiently.

All too common as well is the sad fact that middle-aged and elderly people often misinterpret this condition as the beginning of senile dementia or Alzheimer's disease, and ready themselves for a steady mental and physical decline. Fortunately, much can be done to reverse this condition and renew the ability to think and remember, as you will see as this chapter unfolds.

In comparison with the rest of your body, your brain is a lightweight, about two percent of your total weight. Yet it appropriates about 25 percent of the oxygen you inhale.

Each hour your brain is fueled with about a teaspoon of glucose.

In a remarkable book, *The New Psychiatry*, Nathan Masor, M.D., verifies that the grey matter, where a great deal of your thinking takes place, indeed utilizes as much as 25 percent of your oxygen intake.[1]

Dr. Masor found that the blood in your brain's arteries must have an oxygen saturation of 90 percent for efficient thinking. If it is just 5 percent less (85 percent), your ability for fine concentrating and carrying on precise muscle coordination decreases. Reduce the oxygen saturation to 74 percent, and you start making faulty judgments and decisions. You become emotionally unstable, and your nervous system becomes depressed. Starve yourself of oxygen for four minutes, and you may suffer irreversible brain damage. A little longer than that, and you won't need oxygen, glucose or a doctor—you'll be dead.

Free and Unequal

It's true: We are not all equally endowed physically and mentally. The late Dr. Roger Williams, professor of chemistry and director of the Biochemical Institute at the University of Texas, made this point in one of his landmark books, *Free and Unequal*.[2]

In another book written just a few years later, Dr. Williams indicates that there's a vast variation in size and shapes of different organs. Arteries, too, can be wide or narrow. His analyses of various arteries—and studies by others—reveals this difference.

Mentioning the contrast in size of two arteries coming from the heart's aorta, he writes, "the right subclavian artery has an outside diameter 1.7 times as great as the corresponding artery. It would have roughly three times the cross-section and, therefore, at least three times as much blood-carrying power as the other."[3]

There are extreme variations within us, when compared with other individuals. We all start with different endowments. Some of us have inherited narrow arteries, others wide ones. This fact is especially critical of the carotid artery that feeds blood to our head. Thanks to modern medicine, your doctor can order a test to tell you whether or not your carotid artery is free-flowing or has accumulated biochemical products that limit its diameter. In fact, your doctor can measure blood flow in any major part of your body, enabling you to take appropriate action if necessary.

If you're mentally and physically inactive—if you don't get around much anymore—the blood flow to your brain may become sluggish. But physical and mental inactivity are not the only reasons for the brain becoming oxygen starved and, therefore, inefficient.

Other reasons are low thyroid function (hypothyroidism)—something often overlooked in a doctor's diagnosis—atherosclerosis (partially clogged arteries), every kind of anemia, and certain nutritional deficiencies. Let's consider them one at a time.

The Unsuspected Illness

Before you rule out the possibility of hypothyroidism in your life, please read the following paragraphs. Remember, we mentioned earlier that experts have estimated that up to 40 percent of the population suffers from low thyroid function. Unfortunately this condition is not always detected by conventional lab tests. I was a skeptic about that 40 percent figure early in my medical career when, on my radio interview show, I hosted Broda Barnes, M.D., Ph.D., one of the world's foremost authorities on the thyroid gland.

Dr. Barnes stated that 40 percent of the patients who

came to him turned out to be hypothyroid, challenged physically and mentally. I expressed my doubt at what seemed a preposterous figure, so, in fairness, Dr. Barnes asked me to check it out with my own patients.

I took his advice. And guess what? I quickly shifted from a first-class doubter to a true believer. Slightly more than 40 percent of my patients turned out to be hypothyroid, suffering low energy, cold hands and feet, depression, and difficulty thinking and remembering.

Most of them had been treated by various doctors for their symptoms, rather than for the root cause, and, on natural thyroid supplementation, they experienced amazing reversals of physical and mental health. I began comparing this 40 percent figure with other medical doctor disciples of Dr. Barnes—nearly 100 in all—and their findings were similar to those of Dr. Barnes and me.

The thought of millions of people living fractional lives physically and mentally due to undiagnosed hypothyroidism spurred me to write *Solved: The Riddle of Illness* with my present collaborator, Jim Scheer. Jim was a close friend of Dr. Barnes and, therefore, quite knowledgeable about the thyroid.[4]

Jim and I are thankful that the book—now in its second edition—is a best seller. My files bulge with thank-you letters from people worldwide who benefitted from the book—doctors, too.

Give Your Thyroid Gland Tender Loving Care

Why is the thyroid gland so influential in mind and body? For many reasons. Although a light bow-tie-shaped gland, semicircling the windpipe under the Adam's apple, it exerts an incredibly powerful influence on our lives.

Your five quarts of blood circulate through your thyroid gland every hour, bringing iodide, the substance your thyroid gland needs to make its hormones. Your thyroid gland also stores and discharges thyroid hormone into your bloodstream for delivery to every one of your brain and body cells.

Thyroid hormone sparks metabolism. If the thyroid is under par, it cannot cause proper ignition to create energy in your cells. It's like trying to burn wet wood. There's a lot of smoke but too little fire.

With insufficient thyroid hormone, your heartbeat slows and weakens, blood pressure drops, blood circulation becomes lazy and contributes to discomfort from cold—especially in the hands and feet. Energy and endurance are low, digestion slows down, nails are brittle, wounds heal slowly, the sex urge is weak or dormant, thinking takes effort, and memory is undependable.

Let's hear from the late Louis Berman, M.D., a famous endocrinologist:

"Without thyroid, there can be no complexity of thought, no learning, no education, no habit formation, no responsive energy for situations as well as no physical unfolding of faculty and function. No reproduction of kind with no sign of adolescence at expected age and no exhibition of sex tendencies thereafter."[5]

Can You Pass the Test?

Without the thyroid gland, we would not be human at all. This fact was driven home to me by a new patient of mine, a male computer programmer in his early forties.

"I'm a human vegetable," he told me. "I'm on leave of absence now and doubt whether I can keep my position if I'm ever able to return. I can't think anymore. It's as if I have to push thoughts around in my head physically. And my memory is like a sieve."

His complaints read like a laundry list of hypothyroidism symptoms: being cold all the time, feeling more tired when he awakened in the morning than when he had gone to bed, a blackness of mood and loss of confidence in his ability, and deep depression. I recall when we shook hands upon his arrival that his right hand was so cold it seemed to have been refrigerated.

He was skeptical when I asked him to take the no-cost, at-home, Barnes Basal Temperature Test for thyroid function. "I've taken every imaginable lab test and they all come out as normal. A succession of doctors think I'm a hypochondriac."

"Do me a favor," I replied. "Take the test and come back with the results in three days. I can almost guarantee you'll be on the way to good health in a matter of weeks."

Here's how I instructed him to perform the test.

"Before going to bed tonight, shake down a thermometer and leave it on the bedside table. As soon as you wake up after a good night's sleep—no trip to the bathroom first—tuck the thermometer snugly in your armpit for 10 minutes as you lie there.

"If your thyroid function is normal, your temperature should be in the range from 97.8 to 98.2°F. If it's lower, you may be hypothyroid. Your thyroid gland is under-functioning and your mental and physical problems have probably been caused or at least influenced by that. The test should be done on two consecutive days."

If my patient is a woman of pre-menopausal age, I request that she take the test on the second and third days of her period.

In any event, the computer programmer's test results didn't surprise me. He averaged 95.2. His thyroid blood tests though were borderline normal. I started him out on a quarter grain of natural thyroid supplementation for two weeks. Already by then his morale and energy levels had begun to lift.

Soon I had him on a whole grain of thyroid. A month later, he was renewed in body, mind, and spirit and ready for the back-to-work challenge. I got a kick out of his flash of humor when he expressed his gratitude:

"Thanks, doctor, for unvegetabilizing me." His handshake was much warmer!

The Implications For You

This is not a rare recovery. I have many more in my files, cases in which people were completely restored mentally and physically through a boost to their thyroid gland. Some—first generation hypothyroids—responded simply by taking a 500 mg capsule or tablet of kelp daily. Kelp, a sea vegetable, is one of the best sources of iodine.

Others whose parents and grandparents were hypothyroid usually had to take a small amount of natural thyroid along with nutritional supplements to make themselves equal to daily challenges.

Influence of the thyroid gland comes from more than the spark its hormones provide to combine oxygen and nutrients for mental and physical energy. Thyroid hormone helps determine how powerfully your heart beats—how great the thrust of blood is to reach the extremities: your feet and hands and the tiny capillaries in your brain.

This condition is easily correctable. If you are hypothyroid, however, you must become aware of it in order to do something about it. As you age—let's not blame it solely on added years—and adopt certain harmful lifestyles, your arteries also collect biochemical gunk, narrow down, and limit blood flow.

This is particularly harmful in capillaries so small that blood cells can only move through them in single file. Minor narrowing can make even single-file passage impossible.

Acknowledged as an authority on essential fatty acids (EFAs)—particularly evening primrose oil—David Horrobin, Ph.D., in "Essential Fatty Acids and Aging," explains that a deficiency of EFAs can cause cell walls to become hardened and inflexible.[6]

This deficiency is particularly harmful in red blood cells

that carry oxygen to our brains and throughout our body. Imagine what happens if these cells develop inflexible cell walls.

"Because the diameter of a red cell is greater than the diameter of the capillaries, the red cell must flex in order to pass through easily and to deliver oxygen to the tissue," writes Dr. Horrobin. "Red cell membranes deficient in EFAs become stiffer than normal, do not pass through capillaries so easily and so are likely to lead to reduced tissue oxygenation." (More about this in the next chapter.)

Essential fatty acids are called "essential" because we can't make them in our bodies. We have to *ingest* them in food or supplements. They are also essential as building blocks for cell membranes, hormones, and certain brain neurotransmitters.

Frightening Facts

Let's look at this problem from another standpoint: not cell size or flexibility but diameter of the circulatory vessels. Dr. Nathan Masor states that any narrowing of the key brain arterioles by as small a margin as a sixteenth of an inch can limit the amount of oxygen that gets through, to the point of lowering mental efficiency and bringing on emotional disturbances.[7] In my practice, I use various methods to encourage delivery of oxygen throughout the brain and body: thyroid supplementation to stimulate overall metabolism, a brisk 30-minute walk four to five times weekly—or other regular and vigorous aerobic exercise—for the same purpose and to keep arteries supple and young. I also recommend the heart-strengthening and artery-opening system of Dean Ornish, M.D.

The Ornish system accents eating fresh vegetables, fruit, whole grains, nuts, and seeds. Dr. Ornish then advocates regular aerobic exercise and various ways to prevent and manage stress. Finally, he promotes meditation, a method of taking your mind out of gear to relieve stress.

This program works. Many heart patients have recovered and stimulated vigorous blood circulation through the Ornish system. Some of my patients have also similarly controlled their stress and vastly improved their blood circulation. (See Chapter 8, for more on this subject.)

In the Ornish program it's important to supplement your diet with a multivitamin-mineral—along with calcium, magnesium, and essential fatty acids.

In severe cases of hardening of the arteries, Ornish's therapeutic approach may be supplemented by chelation therapy offered by many M.D.s oriented toward preventive medicine.

Chelation therapy consists of having an intravenous solution containing vitamins, minerals, and EDTA, an FDA approved drug with a 50-year history of safe use, administered by a trained physician over the course of several hours.

Before you undergo chelation therapy, a complete history is taken and a physical exam is performed to make sure your kidneys are healthy and to determine noninvasively how compromised your circulation actually is.

Usually a patient undergoes a course of 20 or more chelation sessions. Hundreds of thousands of successful chelation treatments have been performed in the past 30 years.

The Case of the Dizzy CEO

A successful CEO friend of mine was in such bad shape artery-wise that he became dizzy just from bending to the floor to pick up a pen. It was difficult for him to walk more than fifty paces without rest. And he had to forgo golf, one of his greatest pleasures.

He felt incapable of carrying out his responsibilities. He felt as if he were letting down his employees and shareholders. On the verge of resigning, he came to me. Inasmuch as I do no chelation, I referred him to a physician who does.

After six treatments, his dizzy spells ended. And with each treatment, he felt better and better. Soon he was able to take long walks again. Each day brought him new energy, confidence and problem-solving ability. Twenty-one treatments later, he was a vital CEO again and able to play golf. He was happier than I had seen him in years.

It is oversimplification to say that quality of thinking and remembering depends merely on the efficiency of blood circulation. There's more to it than that: the ability of the bone marrow to make red blood cells, the body's ability to maintain normal temperature, and the size and shape of blood cells for starters.

Red blood cells, for instance, deliver oxygen to the brain and throughout the body for metabolizing food and, through this process, producing energy and heat. If the bone marrow can't make enough red blood cells, the lack will have an impact on how much oxygen is delivered. The result—lower metabolic activity characteristic of hypothyroidism to possibly lower body temperatures generally. Low body temperatures also make it difficult to produce blood cells, as Dr. Barnes discovered in numerous research projects.

Revealing Experiment

Here is a fascinating story told to us by Dr. Barnes that illustrates the importance of normal body temperature.[8]

When Dr. Barnes was a physiology instructor at the University of Chicago many years ago, he witnessed a stunning graphic demonstration. A Ph.D. candidate was puzzled as to why red and white blood cells were formed only in the bone marrow of certain specific bones—the ribs, spine, pelvis and long bones nearest the body. "He suspected that it was a matter of temperature, body organs being warmer than the extremities: arms and legs," Dr. Barnes told us.

To test this hypothesis, he devised a special needle in whose hollow, he inserted a small, thin thermometer to check bone marrow temperature in a white rat.

He found only yellow, non-bloodmaking marrow in the rat's long tail, whose temperature indeed, was lower than that of the blood-producing backbone. Then he curved the rat's tail, made a small incision in the animal's belly, temporarily inserting and suturing the tail there.

Soon the marrow in the tip of the tail, now warmed by the body, was transformed into blood-producing red marrow, while the marrow of the bony structure of the tail's curve remained yellow—unable to make blood cells.

Through some 50 years of practice, this demonstration reminded Dr. Barnes why anemic women often remain pale and depressed, even after having been given extra iron supplement.

Several hundred anemic patients, exhausted and discouraged, regained a more full life when he gave them thyroid supplementation that raised their temperature and increased their body's ability to produce blood cells, especially red corpuscles.

An Iron Supplement May Not Be the Answer

In our practices, Dr. Barnes and I found that supplemental iron therapy is usually only temporarily helpful in the treatment of hypothyroid anemia, because it copes with symptoms, rather than the basic cause that's well-handled by thyroid hormone therapy.

However, it is helpful to some people—certain women of child-bearing years, older infants, children, the elderly, low income groups and minorities—state Robert A. Garrison and Elizabeth Somer in *The Nutrition Desk Reference*. Nor is iron status always discoverable by blood tests, they write. Reduced iron in the blood, in fact, is one of the final stages in iron deficiency.

"For instance, iron is found in the brain as a cofactor in neurotransmitter synthesis. The brain stores are diminished long before blood levels decline."[9]

Foods rich in iron from liver, fish, fowl, meats, fruits, green vegetables, raisins, and brown rice are helpful in individuals with a normal thyroid condition. They are of limited value, however, in a person whose anemia is caused by hypothyroidism.

Body Temperature and Your Brain

Important to note is the fact that a low body temperature common to an underactive thyroid gland can cause brain wave changes that may be misinterpreted by a clinician as neurological damage. In most cases, thyroid therapy will reverse the condition.

Slow reaction time is also common to individuals with low body temperatures characteristic of hypothyroidism. This fact is well documented by accounts of polar explorers subjected to extreme cold who develop hypothermia. Samples of their handwriting while suffering from hypothermia, compared with samples written under normal conditions, show a total lack of coordination.

Body temperatures do not even have to reach such extreme lows to show negative effects on the brain and coordination. Emanuel Donchin, a psychologist, and Noel K. Marshall, an electrophysicist, both of the Cognitive Psychophysiology Laboratory at the University of Illinois, made a significant discovery some years ago. Seemingly small daily changes in body temperature—one or two degrees below normal—reduce certain brain responses in test subjects.[10]

Their findings show that even slightly depressed body

temperatures slow down our movements and higher thought processes. For instance, although we may not even be aware of it, our brains respond more slowly to sound.

Peaks of brain waves have an easily recognizable pattern. If brain wave peaks fail to appear or if they appear later than they should, there's a good possibility of nerve damage. In hypothermia, brain wave peaks are significantly delayed. When temperatures of test subjects are normalized, however, brain wave peaks also speed up to normal.

Donchin and Marshall recommend that medical doctors proceed with caution in diagnosis and consider body temperature of patients before concluding that they have irreversible brain damage. This recommendation is based on their experiments with fifteen test subjects. They discovered that even small temperature changes lowered the efficiency of their subjects' sensory processing, and coordination definitely dropped with their subnormal temperatures and improved markedly when temperatures were raised to normal.

For "Morning" and "Evening" People

Findings of these researchers validate those of G.A. Kerkhof and colleagues at the University of Leiden, Netherlands, who discovered that body temperatures definitely influence the brain in a way that correlates with how subjects rate their performances of various tasks.

Many of us have the tendency to rate ourselves according to work efficiency as "morning" or "evening" people. Kerkhof found that temperatures were normal at peak performance times and lower than normal at other times.

Research of Kerkhof and Donchin and Marshall offer laboratory proof of the handicaps endured by individuals with chronically low body temperatures characteristic of hypothyroidism. Often hypothyroids register temperatures from one to two degrees below normal, as I have observed many times in my own practice.

Frequently, patients with extremely low thyroid function and temperatures to match show the following symptoms: slow motion response, thick-tongued speech, poor coordination, slow mental activity, and impaired memory.

As with low body temperatures, individuals with anemia often manifest lowered ability to think and remember—among upsetting symptoms such as chronic fatigue, pale complexion, being out of breath after minor exertion, high susceptibility to colds and infection, and mild depression.

Earlier we mentioned how narrowed arteries limit the delivery of oxygen-laden blood from the lungs to our trillions of cells. Low quality of hemoglobin (the blood substance that carries the oxygen) can be equally limiting. Each molecule of hemoglobin contains four atoms of iron that make oxygen carrying possible. If there are too few red blood cells or they are too small, they can't deliver enough oxygen.

Are Iron Supplements Necessary?

Iron deficiency anemia is the most common kind of anemia for a variety of reasons: higher than average individual needs for iron, limited ability to absorb iron (usually a matter of insufficient digestive juices, common to the elderly), heavy blood loss—as in injury, surgery, or heavy menstrual flow—and repeated pregnancies, in which the fetus draws a large amount for its own needs.

A diet of heavily processed food—as opposed to fresh food—often supplies too little iron, copper, protein and the vitamins B-6, B-12, folic acid and C necessary for efficient making of hemoglobin. Further, various studies show that a daily intake of from 200 to 500 milligrams of vitamin C can increase iron absorbability immeasurably.

Generally, a diet of unprocessed food can supply all the iron needed, if you consider that all edibles are not created equally. The kind of iron in fish, meat and poultry, called heme, is almost 40 percent absorbed.

The Importance of Being Oxygenated   51

Eggs, dried beans, nuts, and whole grains, along with other nonflesh foods offer a form of iron called ionic. Ionic iron is only about 10 percent absorbed. Vegetarians should be particularly aware of this. Thanks to Popeye the Sailor Man, the myth exists that spinach is a great source of readily available iron, which gave Popeye his legendary strength. Forget it! Just two percent of its ionic iron can be absorbed.

Let me give you a warning about supplemental iron. It's not like a vitamin that's used up. Iron remains in the body and is recycled. Only during stages of growth, pregnancy, menstruation or other blood losses—as in surgery or serious accidents—do we lose an appreciable amount of iron. Infinitesimal amounts of iron exit from the body in sweat, urine, some forms of illness and turnover of cells.

Iron's major task, of course, is twofold: to facilitate the blood's hemoglobin to carry oxygen to the cells and to help the body's proteins to function properly. Any surplus makes the rounds in our bloodstream. When oxidized, this iron converts into free radicals and attacks sound cells.

In extreme cases, excess iron will raise its own danger signal: a bronze discoloration of the skin (a condition called hemochromatosis). In many instances, however, we have no warning of the sabotage taking place underneath: liver injury that could lead to cirrhosis, degeneration marked by the formation of excess connective tissue, and a change in color from healthy red to an unhealthy orange-yellow. So, if you take iron supplementation, do so only with the guidance of a knowledgeable health professional!

Vastly more likely than an iron deficiency in poor thinking and remembering is too little vitamin B–12. A serious deficiency of vitamin B–12 can cause a condition called pernicious anemia. Pernicious means "deadly," and this was an accurate term for this ailment, because pernicious anemia was once fatal.

Early in the twentieth century, the only way to cope with it was by means of blood transfusions. Then three American physicians, led by William P. Murphy, M.D., discovered that eating liver could cure the "incurable." Murphy won the 1934 Nobel prize in medicine for his discovery.[11]

Later, it was found that vitamin B–12 was the prime ingredient in liver that corrected this condition. Confusion, difficulty in thinking, and memory loss are common in extreme pernicious anemia.

The best food sources of vitamin B–12, other than liver, are sardines, mackerel, herring, salmon, lamb, Swiss cheese, eggs, and haddock. Generally we oppose eating canned foods. Canned salmon and sardines, however, are an exception. They offer valuable brain nutrients with the added benefit of bones, an exellent way to keep your own bones strong.

The Unpronounceable Anemia

Still another common form of anemia that undermines thinking and remembering is megaloblastic anemia, a term that indicates malformed red blood cells. A deficiency of both folic acid, found mainly in vegetables and fruit, and vitamin B–12 can cause over-large red blood cells that deliver too little oxygen and sometimes find it difficult to pass through small capillaries in the brain and body.

Usual daily ranges of these vitamins recommended to patients by alternative doctors is 6 to 30 micrograms of vitamin B–12 and 400 micrograms of folic acid.

Clearly, a diet of fresh, unprocessed food with multivitamin and mineral supplementation can be helpful in preventing poor thinking and an undependable memory!

CHAPTER 4

Nutrients That Skyrocket Your I.Q.

The age of giant redwood trees that have been growing for more than a thousand years prompted comedienne Phyllis Diller to remark, "when I want to feel young, I go walking in a grove of redwoods."

If Phyllis really wants to feel young, she should stroll among the ginkgo trees. Some are much older than that!

Botanical Methuselahs themselves, their leaves are something else. For the leaves of the ginkgo tree have a way of keeping our minds young. They can quicken and sharpen our thinking! They can make us forget that we once had a bad memory!

Ginkgo biloba, a substance derived from ginkgo leaves, is truly remarkable. It expands the diameter of our blood vessels and arteries. It fights off damage from free radicals in the brain and throughout the body. It increases the brain's ability to metabolize glucose, stimulates nerve transmission, makes us more mentally alert, increases our attention span, and enhances our ability to think and remember.

Surprise Ending

That's about all it can do for us! Well, not quite. I remember vividly a middle-aged male patient who owned and operated a prosperous, small retail business in a busy mall. He came to me for what he termed "a brain survival kit."

Shaking his head from side to side, he confessed, "Something's drastically wrong. I can hardly think anymore. And my memory is shot. Then there are physical problems, too, but let's deal with my thinking and remembering first."

That's what we did. Results of his Barnes Basal Temperature Test and a blood test showed a near average thyroid gland. So we ruled that out—at least temporarily. My many years of medical experience have shown me that patients whose thyroid seems normal often profit mentally and physically from a small amount of natural thyroid supplementation.

But I did do this: I started him on a 60 milligram ginkgo biloba tablet with breakfast and another in mid-afternoon.

"This will improve the blood circulation in your brain—throughout your body, too. You may or may not notice the difference for three or four weeks, but stay on this regimen for at least several months."

Six weeks later, he phoned my receptionist for an immediate appointment. He urgently needed to see me. On the belief that he had a serious problem, I fitted him into my busy schedule.

It turned out that there was no emergency. He was thrilled. His thinking and remembering had returned.

"I'm so happy," he told me, "and my wife could kiss you."

Before I had a split second to wonder why someone else's wife whom I didn't even know would want to kiss me, he blurted out, "That ginkgo is great stuff. It brought back my mind and *my potency!*"

Wonderful Vitamin B–Complex

Various case histories keep reminding me that some of the old nutritional standbys can work—sometimes work wonders—mentally and physically. I'm talking about a combination of brewer's yeast and desiccated liver that provides an excellent vitamin B–complex.

Why B vitamins? They are important to efficient transport of oxygen inside our brain and body cells. Many of my patients have experienced amazing transformations in mind, spirit, and body from vitamin B–complex.

I suppose rat experiments inspired me about B vitamins. Several studies showed that rats undernourished in the B–complex vitamins have a tougher time thinking their way through a maze than well-nourished ones.

Rats need a minimum of 12½ micrograms of vitamin B–1 daily—among other nutrients—to be well nourished in mind and body. In one particular experiment, when fed only 3 micrograms of this vitamin daily, they were slow in finding their way through a maze. When given 100 micrograms, they hurried through in record time.

That's great for rats, but where's the evidence that vitamin B–1 will help you?

One of the earliest and most dramatic demonstrations of how a nutritional supplement can improve thinking of human beings was achieved with vitamin B–1.

A mixture of curiosity and sharp observation led Dr. Ruth Flinn Harrell to conduct such a study at the Presbyterian Children's Home in Lynchburg, Virginia.[1]

Dr. Flinn Harrell had observed a strange and unanticipated change in a young man, an accident victim, at Johns Hopkins Hospital. Suffering from an aphasia, the loss of ability to speak or write, the patient was going through a long and tedious process of reeducation.

Then, suddenly, he began learning so quickly that he

was healed and able to return to his old job. Intrigued by the rapid recovery, Dr. Flinn Harrell carefully examined case records to find out why. At first she made no headway. Then she noted that for six days before his astonishing recovery, the young man had been given a low potency vitamin B–1 tablet with a meal.

On the trail of something so important, Dr. Flinn Harrell experimented with rats. She tested the maze-solving ability of rats, first with vitamin B–1 added to their diets, then with none. Not suprisingly, she found that vitamin B–1 supplementation enabled the rats to move through the mazes much more quickly.

It Works on Human Beings, Too

Encouraged, Dr. Flinn Harrell decided to try the same vitamin on three children so handicapped that they could not speak. Given a daily vitamin B–complex tablet, all three showed a marked ability to learn. Two actually learned to speak, and then could live a normal life.

Exciting as these findings were, they turned out to be preliminary to the main event. Dr. Flinn Harrell next tested to see if a small amount of vitamin B–1 added to the daily diet could influence the ability to learn, enhance various skills, and even boost I.Q.

In a six-week, double-blind study of paired children and young adults of matched ability—ages 9 to 19—one group was given 2 milligrams of vitamin B–1 daily. The other group was given a look-alike placebo.

Children on the vitamin B–1 scored from 7 to 87 percent higher in mental ability and physical skills than those who took the placebo. The finding led Dr. Flinn Harrell to conclude that a certain nutritional state of the nervous system has to be satisfied for the most effective ability to learn.

Her conclusion was reinforced by results of experiments by two different researchers. Bruno Minz, in the laboratory of the Sorbonne University, Paris, announced in 1938 that a cut nerve leaked a fluid containing vitamin B-1 and, also, that when a nerve was electrically stimulated—as in the human body—it gave off 80 times more vitamin B-1 than a nerve at rest.

During the following year, biochemist R.R. Williams announced that many of the impulses passing through a nerve fiber change that fiber chemically so that it must be constantly supplied with new nutrients through the process of metabolism (fuel burning). Vitamin B-1 appeared to him to help in the burning process.

Modern viewing devices have also revealed that a prolonged deficiency of vitamin B-1 can cause permanent change in brain tissue, making for poor concentration and a faulty memory. Happily, except in instances of extreme neurological damage, thiamin therapy—50 milligrams daily—can bring about dramatic recoveries. It is best to take individual B vitamin fractions such as B-1 with the entire B-complex—50 mg for the major fractions.

The Bell Study: A Forgotten Treasure

Why is taking optimum amounts of vitamin B-1 so important? The answer brings us back to the importance of proper oxidation of brain cells. Thiamine is a key part of a coenzyme system for oxidizing carbohydrates and pyruvic acid, one of several products of carbohydrate oxidation.[2]

A monumental study in the late 1950s accentuates the primary importance of vitamin B-complex—particularly vitamin B-1—in thinking, remembering, and being emotionally sound. Elizabeth C. Bell, Ph.D., surveyed 182 articles, books, and personal communications in writing her lengthy discourse in the *Journal of Psychology*.[3]

Dr. Bell cited the research of D.G. Campbell, from the book *Modern Nutrition in Health and Disease,* who found the brain's neurons (nerves) are more sensitive to changes in nutrition than any other body organ or system. Without vitamin B, carbohydrate foods couldn't be utilized to energize these nerves.

Another study cited by Dr. Bell involved mental patients. Researchers drastically reduced their intake of vitamin B–1 far below the needed level for 147 days. Within 10 days to two weeks, the patients were unable to concentrate, their thinking was confused, they could remember little, and they were pysically weak and depressed.

All of them were irritable with explosive tempers erupting at the slightest provocation, quarrelsome, depressed, and under a black cloud of impending doom. Two threatened suicide.

Also cited in the Elizabeth Bell study was research by Dr. Tom Spies, quoted as follows:

"Most malnourished patients have some degree of mental disturbance which frequently is the only evidence of anything wrong early in the story."

Spies also indicated that, under such circumstances, wrong diagnoses are more than possible—for instance, hysteria, depression, or anxiety state. Inasmuch as these symptoms can be caused by dietary deficiencies, Dr. Spies turned them around within 30 minutes to 20 hours with vitamin B–1 or the entire vitamin B–complex, plus a substantial diet of natural and whole foods.

How Not to Short-Change Your Mind

It is a sin of neglect and omission that the Elizabeth Bell study is gathering dust, rather than attracting the attention of doctors. The difficulty many patients have in thinking and remembering could be turned around with B complex vitamins added to a sound diet. Too bad that present-day researchers and society worship the new—even if not sufficently tried—and neglect the old and tried!

Nutrients That Skyrocket Your I.Q.

Sadly, many Americans fail to take in enough vitamin B–1 and are draining away their low supply without being aware of it. In brief, they are short-changing their mind—their body, too—and falling far below their potential to think.

Are you among them? Test yourself to see if you're sabotaging your mind in the following ways:

1. Do you eat white bread and refined and processed cereals regularly?
2. Do you add sugar to your cereals or beverages and eat candy or pastries every day?
3. Do you have one or more alcoholic drinks daily without taking a vitamin B–complex supplement?
4. Do you smoke regularly?
5. Do you eat cooked vegetables most of the time?
6. Do you eat raw fish frequently?
7. Do you drink two or more cups of coffee daily?
8. Are you on the Pill? Are you pregnant or nursing?
9. Do you take antacids after one or more daily meals?
10. Are you stressed at work, at home, with a chronic physical ailment, anxiety or deep depression?
11. Do you take estrogen or sulfa drugs?

If you answered "yes" to three or more of these questions, you may be vitamin B–1 deficient. The more "yesses," the more the possible deficiency.

Here's a list of food supplements and foods richest in vitamin B–1, in terms of milligrams per 100 grams, just under four ounces.

Brewer's yeast	16
Torula yeast	15
Sunflower seeds	2.2
Wheat germ	2.0
Royal jelly[1]	1.5

Pine nuts	1.3
Peanuts[2]	1.2
Soybeans	1.1
Sesame seeds	0.98
Brazil nuts	0.96
Bee pollen	0.93
Pecans	0.86
Alfalfa and Peas	0.80
Millet	0.73
Buckwheat and Oats	0.60
Hazelnuts	0.46
Rye	0.43
Lentils and Corn	0.37

(1) Royal Jelly is a super-food, a thick, white, milky substance which worker bees feed to the Queen Bee to turn her into a magnificent specimen able to lay as many as 2,000 eggs daily and live many times longer than other bees. It contains the entire vitamin B complex, with a high concentration of pantothenic acid—the antistress vitamin—as well as vitamins A, C, D, E, enzymes, hormones, 18 amino acids and antibacterial substances.

(2) Peanuts are sometimes contaminated with aflatoxin, a mold that can cause cancer. Therefore, they should not be eaten frequently. Despite limitation of aflatoxin levels by government standards, peanuts still contain too much, state many experts. In Third World countries where peanuts are eaten frequently, the incidence of liver cancer is high. It is best to eat peanuts—other nuts, too—without salt.

Brown rice	0.34
Walnuts	0.33
Egg yolk	0.32
Chickpeas	0.31
Blackstrap molasses	0.28
Liver	0.25
Almonds	0.25
Barley	0.21
Salmon	0.21
Eggs	0.17

Lamb	0.15
Mackerel	0.15

Over and above vitamin B–1 rich foods, some of my patients wish to guarantee themselves maximum brain power by taking a vitamin B–1 supplement. However, as stated earlier, I recommend that they take a vitamin B–complex tablet or capsule containing 50 to 100 milligrams (mg) of the major B fractions daily, because taking one member of the family daily for a long period can sometimes cause imbalances.

Of course, the vitamin B–complex tablet or capsule works better if you eat mainly whole grain cereals and bread, raw or lightly cooked vegetables; minimize or eliminate coffee, alcohol, and smoking; and learn to handle stressors as challenges you can cope with, rather than as overwhelming depressants, frustrations or obstacles you can't cope with.

Dr. Tom Spies: A Man for the Ages

Early in my medical career, I was deeply impressed with the pioneering research that gave revealing insights to the late Tom Spies, M.D., who was instrumental in launching a school of nutrition at Northwestern University Medical College in Evanston, Illinois—a rarity in medical colleges. I remain impressed.[4]

In the mid-1950s, it was still fashionable to believe that infectious disease caused pellagra, rampant in the southern United States. Pellagra drained the body of energy, invited a host of physical and emotional problems, and slowed thinking processes.

Dr. Spies traced pellagra to a deficiency of niacin, one of the B vitamins. Processed corn was a staple in the diet—especially among poor people. Unfortunately, this grain lacks the amino acid lysine and contains a limited amount of another amino acid called tryptophan. The milling process removed most of the tryptophan. This is significant, because tryptophan is changed into niacin in the body.

Dr. Spies upgraded the diets of pellagra sufferers to include more B–complex and supplemented their diet with niacin. Almost miraculously, his patients at Hillman Hospital in Birmingham, Alabama, recovered.

They became energized. Their anxiety, depression, hysteria, jitteriness, restlessness, tension, or nervousness disappeared. Their soreness of mouth and tongue left. Their aversion to bright lights and bright colors and noises disappeared.

"I could not accept the concept that their brains were irreparably damaged," wrote Dr. Spies. "It seemed that the brain cells were waiting listlessly and would function again at full efficiency when we gave them the required nutrients."

He made an astonishing discovery. On the new dietary regimen, the patients showed a change in the content of lactose (sugar) and lactic acid entering and leaving their brains. Dr. Spies found that in patients deficient in B–complex vitamins—particularly niacin—there was a 60 percent decrease in brain metabolism, the rate at which the brain uses oxygen and nutrients for energy. Imagine what happens to a brain operating at 40 percent efficiency.[5]

Consuming as little as 50 milligrams of niacin with every meal for several days reversed patients from being depressed and fearful to being cheerful and courageous. Slow thinking, mental fogginess, and a poor memory disappeared almost magically.[6]

A reminder: If you're taking an individual vitamin B family member, don't forget to back it up with vitamin B–complex.

Glutamic Acid: Brain Fuel

Here is another significant discovery with another nutrient. Almost a generation ago, on a hunch, three researchers at the Columbia College of Physicians and Surgeons conducted a study that led to the discovery of an important brain-enhancer.[7]

Drs. Zimmerman, Burgemeister, and Putnam knew that glutamic acid, an amino acid, is one of two forms of "fuel" that the brain uses for developing needed energy. Shouldn't it have some influence on thinking ability? They set out to find the answer.

First, they fed concentrated amounts of glutamic acid to rats. Those on glutamic acid thought their way through a maze twice as fast as rats not given this supplement.

This result encouraged them to determine if glutamic acid would rev up the I.Q. of 69 mentally retarded children and youths, ages 5 to 17, whose I.Q.s averaged 65.

For a year these children, all volunteers, were given 12 grams of glutamic acid daily with their food, a large amount because this nutrient has difficulty crossing the blood–brain barrier. Sure enough, the average gain in their I.Q. was 11 points, with some rising as high as 17 points.

Their problem-solving ability dramatically improved, along with their personalities and ability to relate to others. When glutamic acid was no longer administered, they all suffered a sharp decline in I.Q.

Knowing that the amide form of glutamic acid crosses the blood–brain barrier more readily than glutamic acid, the late Dr. Roger Williams, the biochemist who isolated pantothenic acid, also studied its effects on mentally retarded children.

Associates of Williams, Drs. Lorene Rogers and Ross B. Pelton, tested effects of the amino acid L-glutamine on these children, again volunteers. This supplement raised their I.Q.s to a significant level.[8]

And for adults? Dr. Williams recommends 1,000 to 4,000 milligrams. It is impossible to derive this much from normal amounts of food. A harmless natural substance, L-glutamine is available in tablet or capsule form in health food stores.[9]

Dr. Wurtman Shatters a Myth

Here's a cliche that's old enough to be retired on Social Security: "You are what you eat." Too bad it isn't retired, because it's inaccurate and incomplete. You are also what you *don't* eat. There are dietary sins of omission as well as commission. Furthermore, what you eat and what you don't eat influence your mind as well as your body.

Until numerous breakthroughs and revelations by Dr. Richard Wurtman, biochemist at the Massachusetts Institute of Technology, medical students were fed the fiction that "if you give the brain its quota of glucose and oxygen, it will make whatever else it needs." This was supposed to be true regardless of the nutrition given the body and your efficiency—or lack of it—in metabolizing nutrients.

Thankfully, this belief was shattered by Dr. Wurtman and MIT associates. Numerous Wurtman experiments proved conclusively that what you ate for breakfast, lunch, or dinner influences how efficiently neurons (nerve cells) in your brain function.

Neurotransmitters, of course, are the chemical messengers that fire signals from one nerve cell to others with lightning speed. If you are not eating enough of the right foods, your brain may not make neurotransmitters quickly and well enough to meet demand. So your thinking may not reach peak performance.[10]

When Dr. Edith Cohen, a member of the Wurtman team, fed large amounts of the B vitamin choline to lab rats, the quantity of the neurotransmitter acetylcholine increased in them.[11]

Later the Wurtman team found that choline-containing lecithin, a substance derived from egg yolk, milk, soybeans, and corn, produced greater amounts of choline in the blood than did choline itself. The high level of choline also lasted much longer than it did when test subjects ate choline itself.

Eat Your Way to Mental Alertness

A fascinating discovery by Wurtman and company is that if you eat a meal accenting protein—like eggs, meat or fish—you are far more mentally alert than if you eat a meal high in carbohydrates, such as fruits and vegetables and cereals.

The latter will reduce your thinking efficiency and make you sleepy—hardly a desirable state in this highly competitive world. Why is this? An essential amino acid—one your body can't make—tryptophan is difficult to absorb and take into the brain.

Found in turkey and milk, with lesser amounts in brown rice, lentils, peanuts, pumpkin, and sesame seeds, tryptophan has difficulty making it into the brain. It seems that other amino acids fill the seats of the transport system first. With a high carbohydrate meal, however, tryptophan has less competition from other amino acids and gets through.

Wurtman and associates found that the amount of tryptophan in the brain and blood plasma determines the amount of serotonin, a neurotransmitter in the brain. The latter induces tranquility and sleepiness and reduces sensitivity to pain.

Formerly that warm glass of milk recommended by many doctors to invite sleep was thought to achieve this purpose due to its high calcium content. Now researchers are divided. Many feel that tryptophan is the content of concern here. A deficiency of several other well-known nutrients can also handicap thinking—vitamin A and zinc, for example.

Some years ago, a team of Indonesian biochemists set out to test the validity of the widely held belief that undernutrition in infancy and early childhood can cause irreversible damage to the mind.[12]

Led by Pek Hien Liang, M.S., and Tijook Tiauw Hie, M.D., the team measured the intelligence of 107 children from age 5 to 12. Forty-six of them had been classified as malnourished, 17 with symptoms of vitamin A deficiency. The others were rated as healthy.

The team studied the children's intelligence through clinical and biochemical examinations, including a focus on food intake. For greater validity, examiners in the research department at the University of Indonesia gave the children intelligence tests.

The group that had manifested symptoms of vitamin A deficiency and other indications of malnutrition made the lowest I.Q. scores. One of the most interesting aspects of the study was a joint observation by the team. Intellectual and physical development of the children "could be predicted with a high degree of accuracy on the basis of their nutritional status during the pre-school years."

The team concluded their findings this way: children who had been malnourished showed the lowest I.Q.s, while children who had never been diagnosed as malnourished showed the highest I.Q.

Good Nutrition in Early Years Is Important

Similar findings resulted from a study of monkeys by Mari Golub, a behavioral biologist at the University of California, Davis, primate research center. To determine the types of mental and physical problems that might occur in zinc-deprived human beings, Golub and associates studied rhesus monkeys whose human development and metabolism are similar to those of people.[13]

Following 10 monkeys from birth through their adolescent growth spurt, the researchers gave half of the group 100 parts per million of zinc daily—considerably more than required. The other half were given just four parts per million of zinc daily in the womb and after delivery. They termed this a "marginal zinc deprivation."

The zinc-deprived monkeys showed zinc blood levels 38 percent lower than those of the other group, a depressed immune function, and obvious learning impairment. In one of several tests, the zinc-deficient monkeys took two to three times as long to learn the difference between a circle and a cross.

Similar rat experiments produced the same results, leading Dr. Harold Sandstead, of the University of Texas Medical Branch in Galveston, to comment that problems are arising in developing countries where malnourished individuals are just getting by on a low zinc diet: vegetables, cereals, and no meat.[14]

In the book *Future Youth,* Roy Hullin, M.D., is also paraphrased to the effect that zinc helps to activate at least 80 nervous system enzymes involved in the thinking process. In a study of 1200 patients over age 55, Dr. Hullin discovered that the 220 senile individuals among them had significantly lower blood levels of zinc than those who were not senile.[15]

In an animal study, two Texas researchers, Elizabeth Root, Ph.D., and John Longenecker, found that deficiencies of two other common nutrients—the trace mineral copper and vitamin B-6—can cause devastating mental results.[16]

There's more to this than just making sure you have ingested 2 milligrams of copper daily. Zinc and copper compete for the same absorption sites in the small intestine. Excessive amounts of zinc can crowd out copper. A generally agreed-upon ratio for copper to zinc is 2 milligrams to 25–30 milligrams. The multipurpose mineral formulas that you can buy at your local vitamin store usually have an acceptable ratio for these trace minerals.

Earlier we observed that not stimulating and challenging the brain—living a no-brainer vegetative life—can lead to a shrinkage of dendrites, those tiny treelike appendages that carry electrical impulses from one brain cell to another. Now the Texas biochemists find that deficiencies in zinc and vitamin B–6 can also cause dendrites to shrivel and die. Something similar can happen to human beings deficient in these nutrients, say the researchers.

Sure Your Vitamin C Intake Is High Enough?

In numerous human studies, insufficient vitamin C has been associated with poor problem-solving ability. And this is the vitamin known mainly for promoting healthy blood vessels, gums, teeth, and bones; for shortening the duration of colds and flu; for accelerating wound-healing; and for strengthening the immune system.

Vitamin C, however, has a little-known but essential function in the central nervous system (CNS), including the brain and spinal cord. The central nervous system is the most important part of the body.

There's no organ or area of the body that contains more unsaturated fats than the CNS. This makes it a prime target for attack by free radicals. As vitamin C is one of the most powerful antioxidants and free radical fighters, nature endowed us with what we call a vitamin pump. The pump actually has two parts. One part draws vitamin C out of circulating blood and then concentrates this vitamin by 10 times in the spinal fluid.[17]

The second part draws vitamin C out of the spinal fluid, concentrates it still more—by a factor of 10 times—and drives it to surround and bathe the nerve cells of the spinal cord and the brain with a total concentration 100 times greater than in any other body fluids.

Several research projects show that vitamin C can boost the I.Q. For example, one project revealed that matched students with high blood serum levels of vitamin C had an

I.Q. almost five points higher than those with lower blood levels of this vitamin.[18]

This doesn't sound like much of a margin, but the researchers pronounced it "statistically significant." Then both groups were given additional vitamin C—a glass of orange juice daily for six months. The group that had shown a superior I.Q. level gained only 1/100 of a point, but the other group gained 3.54 points.

These are some of the contributions to better thinking and greater brain health that the nutrients familiar to us can make. There are also some spectacular results from supplements that are less familar to us. This is the subject of the next chapter!

CHAPTER 5

Brain Transplant or Something Better?

One of my favorite patients, a white-haired, retired stockbroker who's always good for a laugh, came into my offices concerned about a slowdown in his thinking and his "sieve-like memory."

"Dr. Langer, I want a brain transplant," he said.

You don't play this fellow straight, so I replied: "Do you want it done in my office or in the parking lot?"

There are less drastic ways of achieving my patient's objectives. Several of the lesser known nutrient supplements offer effective, practical, low-cost ways to sharpen thinking and remembering. One of the best is phosphatidylserine (fos-fa-tie-dyl-SEER-ine), a hard to pronounce but easy to take supplement.

So many of my patients have had brain revivals from phosphatidylserine (PS) that I know it can't be coincidence.

A phosphorus-containing fat, this substance is essential for healthy cell membranes throughout the body and brain. It helps cell membranes stay flexible for the easy entry of oxygen and nutrients and the exit of wastes. Almost 60 percent of our brain is fat, which is desperately needed to produce and transmit electrical energy.

The body usually makes sufficient phosphatidylserine until middle-age or beyond, when we need it most. Then due to nutritional deficiencies, wear and tear of negative lifestyles, and accumulated stresses, production slows down. So does our thinking and remembering.

However, supplementation with PS renews cell membrane flexibility and flushes away accumulated wastes. Dr. Robert Atkins colorfully characterizes PS as "a biological brain detergent" that creates more receptors on brain cells (upgrading communication between nerve cells), corrects stress-related nerve damage, and recharges the ability to think and remember.[1]

It has proven helpful in upgrading the performance of patients with Parkinson's disease and Alzheimer's disease.

Need More Convincing?

More than 30 studies reveal that supplemental PS can improve learning ability and thinking power. One of the most convincing, that of Thomas Crook, M.D., and associates, dealt with 149 volunteers above 50 years old. Over 12 weeks, about half of the total took 100 milligrams of PS three times daily. The other half of the group took placebos.[2]

Results surprised even the research team. Those on phosphatidylserine demonstrated a sensational gain of 15 percent in learning and remembering. The best news of all: The most impaired individuals showed the most dramatic gains. Gains by the placebo takers were negligible.

A key research team member had no hesitation in announcing that PS apparently reversed roughly 12 years of mental decline!

Most PS supplements are derived from soy lecithin. Although their cost can stress the wallet or purse—roughly around $100 per month for 100 mg three times daily—results make it all worthwhile. It's next to impossible to derive enough PS by ingesting soy lecithin. That would mean eating prodigious amounts at a prohibitive cost.

For those on a tight budget, however, I recommend the individual nutrients from which PS is made in the body: the sulfur-containing amino acid methionine, essential fatty acids, folic acid, and vitamin B−12.

Foods richest in methionine are eggs, fish, liver, milk, whole grains, corn, nuts, rice, and seeds. (I also recommend going easy on alcoholic drinks, which are known for destroying methionine.) Folic acid (from the Latin "folium," meaning "leaf") comes mainly from green vegetables and other plant tissues.

Essential fatty acids include the Omega-6 series found in linoleic acid and the Omega−3 series derived from linolenic acid. They are as necessary to health and well-being as vitamins and minerals.

The Omega−6 fatty acids are found mainly in soy, sunflower seeds, corn, wheat germ, and walnuts. Omega−3 fatty acids are derived principally from fish, flaxseeds, and chia seeds, among others.

Chia is an ancient wonder food used by the Aztecs in pre-Columbian times and Native Americans in the Southwest. It is known for imparting high energy and endurance. Until recently as well, because it grew wild and was difficult to harvest, there was never enough of a supply to meet the demand in health food stores. Now it has been domesticated and will soon be available to everyone. Chia contains a favorable ratio of Omega−3 to Omega−6—approximately 6 to 4.

Although both Omega−3 and Omega−6 fatty acids are necessary, it is possible to ingest too much Omega−6 with some negative health consequences.

The best approach is to make sure you eat more Omega−3-rich cold-water fish several times a week—halibut, salmon, mackerel. This practice can help tilt the teeter-totter in favor of Omega−3. Flaxseed oil and chia are best sources of the latter.

All oils are perishable—sensitive to heat and light—and become rancid easily. All flaxseed and chia oil should be sold in black bottles and stored in a cool dark place or refrigerated. They should be used quickly.

For its part, gamma–linolenic acid, a versatile nutrient, produces prostaglandins—short-term regulators of body function—and has a good track record for coping with arthritis, diabetes, skin eruptions, and multiple sclerosis. Although it can be evolved from Omega–6 oil, it must struggle through a veritable biochemical obstacle course first. This process ranges from difficult to impossible. Some of the obstacles are a diet heavy in saturated fats, alcohol intake, use of processed oils and foods, additives to foods, zinc deficiency, the aging process, degenerative diseases, virus infections, and exposure to radiation.

Your best bet here is to ingest gamma–linolenic acid in evening primrose oil—8 to 9 percent GLA—borage oil or black currant seed oil. Richest sources of vitamin B–12 are liver, kidney, fish, eggs, and beef.

Please note that fish appears on three of the four above lists. That's why I recommend it as a two to three times a week entree, along with daily green salads made from fresh, crisp vegetables. This lower cost way of buying the source ingredients for PS has helped my patients.

Ginkgo: The Wonder Worker

Although we mentioned ginkgo biloba as a brain-booster in the previous chapter, it is worth mentioning again, because it does much more for efficient thinking than increase blood flow.

Receptors on the surface of brain cells decrease in number as we age, and their ability to bind neurotransmitters decreases, too; so, transmission of brain impulses slows down.

When ginkgo biloba was fed to old rats in a study by biochemist F. Huguet, they secreted more noradrenaline, and their ability to bind neurotransmitters increased by 28 percent.[3]

Another exciting brain product is dimethylaminoethanol—DMAE for short—a source of choline that's storable in infinitesimal amounts in brain neurons. It tends to disappear as we age. DMAE increases I.Q., attention span, and ability to learn and remember. It helps to correct hyperactivity—attention deficit disorder, if you prefer—in children. Anchovies and sardines are the richest sources of DMAE.

Inasmuch as few of us can eat sardines or Caesar salads daily—or take our anchovies straight—it's a challenge to derive much DMAE from foods. DMAE supplements, however, can help.

There are two theories as to how DMAE works. One is that it speeds up the brain's synthesis and turnover of a key neurotransmitter, acetylcholine, essential to thinking. Two is that it blocks the metabolism of choline in body tissues, increasing the amount of this nutrient entering the brain and stimulating brain cell receptors.

Whether you believe in theory one or two, there's full agreement that it revs up mental processes. Reporting in *Clinical Pharmacology and Therapeutics,* H.B. Murphree and associates, showed by experiment that DMAE solves an acute problem of seniors of advanced age: inability to pay attention (key to learning) and to concentrate on writing and studying. It also encourages quicker and better sleep.[4]

Don't Overlook DMAE and Acetyl-L-Carnitine!

DMAE brought about an impressive improvement in Attention Deficit Disorder in 25 girls and 83 boys in a study by the late Dr. Carl Pfeiffer, of the Brain Bio Center in

Princeton, New Jersey. More than 60 percent of the boys and 75 percent of the girls showed positive improvements in learning and behavior problems here.[5]

A greater attention span, decreased irritability, and a noticeable gain in the ability to learn, even, in certain instances, an increase in I.Q. showed why DMAE is an important supplement to take.

Another noteworthy brain enhancer, acetyl-L-carnitine, heightens our natural capacity to transport fat across cell membranes so that the energy furnaces in each cell, or mitochondria, have more fuel to burn. Acetyl-L-carnitine carries out the same functions as plain carnitine, the body's own substance, but does them better.

It energizes the brain, slows its aging, and protects brain cells from free radical damage. Ward Dean, M.D., John Morgenthaler and Stephen Fowkes, in *Smart Drugs: The Next Generation,* cite two Italian studies. One shows that an acetyl-L-carnitine supplement improves the mental performance of young and healthy people, as well as that of middle-agers and above who are losing their ability to synthesize this nutrient.[6]

Seventeen volunteers were fed 1500 milligrams of acetyl-L-carnitine or a placebo daily for 30 days. Prior to the study, they were tested for attention levels, hand-eye coordination, and for reflexes.

Those on acetyl-L-carnitine showed increased speed of reflexes compared with the others, completing their test tasks three to four times faster with a far lower rate of error.

In another Italian study, half of 236 mentally impaired elderly people were given 1,500 milligrams of acetyl-L-carnitine daily and the other half, a look-alike placebo. After five months, those on acetyl-L-carnitine improved markedly in ability to think, remember, and achieve a relaxed state.[7] Unlike the positive benefits gained from many other nutrients, those from acetyl-L-carnitine persist long after supplementation stops.

Unexpected Benefits

In considering supplements that enhance thinking, two of my favorites are real sleepers: evening primrose oil and garlic. Used by Native Americans for hundreds of years, evening primrose oil is pressed from the seeds of a lovely, yellow Eastern Seaboard wildflower that blooms and dies in a single evening. Its oil contains nine percent gamma–linolenic acid (GLA), an essential fatty acid that is virutally nonexistent in the American diet.

Theoretically, at least, GLA can be derived from linoleic acid, but it also must survive a veritable biochemical obstacle course to become gamma–linolenic acid. Diets heavy in saturated fats and cholesterol, processed vegetable oil and alcohol are impediments, along with aging and slower metabolism, virus infections, degenerative diseases, radiation and zinc deficiency.

Gamma–linolenic acid is the substance from which the body makes a family of hormonelike compounds called prostaglandins (PGs) that exercise short-term control over every organ in the body. (Their name brings to mind the prostate gland, where they were first discovered.)

These prostaglandins have much to do with preventing abnormal clotting of blood, poor circulation, heart disease, and a weak immune system.

In his booklet, *Evening Primrose Oil,* Richard Passwater, Ph.D., makes this pertinent statement about gamma–linolenic acid:

"Anyone deficient in GLA will also have a shortage of prostaglandins, resulting in impaired health. The nutritional optimization of PG is a revolutionary breakthrough in health care."[8] (Remember that GLA is also present in borage oil and black currant seed oil.)

Abnormal blood clotting or irregular heartbeat can cause a blockage of blood flow, or spasms of a critical artery—

in a phrase, a heart attack. Without enough blood, heart tissue dies.

Usually blood is slippery so that it can flow freely inside smooth arteries. When we cut ourselves, the blood automatically starts its clotting. Platelets half the size of red blood cells become sticky and adhere to one another.

A healthy person has what's called a platelet adhesion index around 20. Often this index rockets up to 90 for heart attack victims. Artery linings make a substance called prostacyclin (PGI2) that keeps blood platelets from sticking to them or to one another. Arteries lined with layers of fat, cholesterol, calcium, and ceroids or damaged by high blood pressure, however, can't make prostacyclin; so, more biochemical materials collect and narrow the arteries.

This is where evening primrose oil comes in. Its gamma–linolenic acid makes the prostaglandin (PGE1) that keeps the blood slippery and more able to penetrate the narrow conduits to the brain and elsewhere.

My patients protect against arterial blockage, heart attacks, and strokes with two 500 mg evening primrose capsules daily.

The Sweet Smell of Success

Now how does garlic fit in? Garlic is what I call a "do everything nutrient." It helps assure the brain a steady supply of oxygen-rich blood. It prevents blood fats from sticking to artery walls. It lowers blood pressure to protect against strokes and heart attacks and blocks the body from releasing a substance called thromboxane B–2 that causes blood vessels to constrict.

Bonus values from garlic include stimulating the immune system, coping with infectious diseases, decreasing elevated blood sugar, and raising metabolism so that some patients can lose unwanted weight.

I encourage patients to take odorless, aged, high potency garlic capsules, at least 1,000 milligrams daily, and to eat garlic as a seasoning in various foods.

Controversy does exist though about a certain aspect of processed, deodorized garlic. One camp claims that the ingredient allicin is most important. The other camp says it's not that important.

It's when you crush raw garlic that you get allicin. Unfortunately, the allicin doesn't last. Further, most of the studies showing garlic's merit in prevention or cure praise aged, odorless, garlic organically grown. So my vote goes to odorless, aged garlic.

My patients are delighted with the latter and are so healthy in mind, body and spirit that they rarely come back to me for treatment. And that's the way it should be. Doctors are supposed to cure people, not keep them coming back. So hooray for all the nutrients mentioned earlier and for evening primrose oil and garlic! They used to be my secret weapons for helping patients. No more though; knowledge of their curative properties now belongs to you, too!

CHAPTER 6

CATS and Your Mind

A noted specialist in environmental medicine, James Braly, M.D., of Encino, California, warns against CATS because of what they can do to your health.

It's not the furry, purring, sleeping-in-the-sun pets that he's talking about, although they can cause allergies in certain susceptible people. Dr. Braly is referring to the acronym "CATS" that stands for Coffee, Alcohol, Tobacco, and Sugar.[1]

Let's start with first things first, that steaming, wake-up cup of morning coffee. Is Dr. Braly saying that there are sufficient grounds for divorcing ourselves from coffee?

Not at all. He merely wants to make us aware of the pros and cons of coffee and its super-stimulating ingredient, caffeine, the most popular central nervous system stimulant. H.L. Newbold in *Dr. Newbold's Nutrition for Your Nerves* makes this confession[2]: "I hate to disillusion you, but like every other person in the world, I lack perfection. (Please don't tell anyone!) I have a cup of black coffee first thing in the morning...."

I also have a cup of black coffee in the morning to get

the motor started! Jim Scheer, my collaborator, starts his motor with a cup of black coffee in the morning, too.

Dr. Richard Wurtman and associates in the Department of Brain and Cognitive Sciences at M.I.T.—as well as other researchers—find low to moderate amounts of caffeine helpful: 32 to 256 milligrams daily. Caffeine in a cup of coffee ranges from about 80 to 120 milligrams, as reported in a *Medical Tribune News Service* article.[3]

Caffeine can rev up alertness and mood, significantly enhance performance in word association challenges, and decrease reaction time. German researchers have also found that caffeine speeds up reading without increasing errors.

Still other investigators have found that caffeine increases attention span and ability to concentrate, hones mental sharpness, enhances accuracy with numbers, and heightens auto driving skills.

On the other side of the ledger, caffeine can increase blood pressure and can bring on irregular heartbeat, irritability, jumpiness, stomach upsets, panic attacks, and sleeplessness.

A Safe Limit to Coffee Drinking?

Researchers generally agree that the caffeine in two cups of coffee daily—roughly 200 milligrams—is not harmful. Nonsmokers who drink up to three cups of coffee daily may experience a small rise in systolic and diastolic blood pressure, but this tends to recede after several days—a week at most. Such intake plus the nicotine from regular smoking, however, may elevate blood pressure to a dangerous level.

Those in whom caffeine causes irregular heartbeat, what one writer characterizes as "crazy rhythm," had better cut down on caffeine or cut it out. Hair-trigger irritability, explosive temper, panic attacks, and difficulty falling asleep or staying that way are all warnings that may indicate too great an intake of caffeine.

A review of coffee studies for the past 10 years tells us that up to three cups daily seems safe for most people. Some studies do show that coffee can remove the mineral potassium from your system—even to creating a deficiency.

Various other studies indicate that four or more cups of coffee daily can make calcium absorption less efficient and may even cause abnormal amounts of this mineral to be lost in the urine.

One overlooked nutritional reduction caused by caffeine is that of vitamin B–1, even though a gram of coffee contains 10 milligrams of this vitamin.

It is a mistake to calculate your intake of caffeine strictly in terms of amount of coffee drunk, as I tell my patients. There's caffeine in most soft drinks, nonherbal teas, cocoa, and chocolate. Further, cocoa and chocolate contain still another stimulant, theobromine—to 1 to 2 percent of its total volume. Considering its theobromine content, a large chocolate candy bar would have the stimulating effect of a cup of coffee.

I discourage my patients from substituting soft drinks for coffee, even though some of them are caffeine- and sugarfree, because the safety of sugar substitutes used in them has not been established to my satisfaction. Then, too, soft drinks contain phosphoric acid. If several cans or bottles are consumed in a day, the intake of phosphorus could outweigh that of calcium, creating an unfavorable balance and a loss of calcium needed to assure us of a lifetime of sound and sturdy bones.

Caffeine is often richly present in various over-the-counter drugs: cold remedies, painkillers, stimulants, and weight control products. Caffeine is often present, but not mentioned, in prescription drugs as well.

Two Sides to the Alcohol Story

There's bad and good news about another one of the CATS, alcohol. First the bad news. In winter some years ago, I got the shock of my life. I attended an autopsy on an alcoholic who froze to death while in a drunken stupor on a New York City street.

When his skull was opened for examination, there was actually no brain structure at all—only a mass of mush. That's what alcohol and malnutrition had done. This is the reason why medical schools cannot use the brains of chronic alcoholics for teaching purposes.

That experience is one of the prime reasons I wanted to write this book—as an exhibit of what alcoholism can do to a perfectly good brain.

With so much information released about how a drink or two of alcohol daily can help to prevent heart disease, another side of the story should be told: the negative effects of even moderate amounts of intoxicants.

Unexplained strokes and hemorrhages that sometimes affect the thinking and memory now have a rational explanation. So says a team of investigating physiologists at the State University of New York's Downstate Medical Center in Brooklyn.[4]

Such disorders occur within 24 hours after heavy drinking. Usually less than an ounce of alcohol causes spasms of arterioles—branches of arteries slightly larger than capillaries—and cuts off oxygen, a condition called hypoxia. This reaction is exactly what happens in strokes.

The findings of this research team also explain why alcohol brings on blackouts, brain damage, and hallucinations, among other psychiatric problems.

Reduced oxygen in the brain and body first produces euphoria, fuzzy-mindedness, and verbal play. Then with more alcohol and more pronounced spasms of brain arterioles, come somewhat impaired vision, poor muscle coordination, slurred speech, unsteadiness, and staggering. The next stage brings coma, stupor, and episodes resembling strokes.

Arteriole constriction at this point can be extreme enough to choke off oxygen-laden blood and damage brain cells or networks of them, either temporarily or permanently. Stroke can occur when the damage covers a large enough area.

A Biography of Strokes

Blockages of blood flow, due to a series of spasms, can also elevate blood pressure. If the alcohol intake is high and frequent, arteriole walls may weaken and, under extreme pressure, rupture. Consequently, chronic alcoholics experience a high rate of strokes, extremely high blood pressure, and sudden death while on a binge, explain the researchers.

Validation of this study comes from another source, research conducted at Dudley Road Hospital in Birmingham, England, and at various institutions in the United States.

The English researchers interviewed 230 stroke patients about their drinking habits and compared them with other age- and sex-matched patients hospitalized for reasons other than stroke and alcohol use. Here's what they found.

Weekly drinking of more than 300 grams of alcohol, roughly 30 drinks, made men four times more prone to suffer strokes than nondrinkers. Light drinkers—one to nine drinks a week—showed only half the stroke risk of nondrinkers.

Heavy drinking has been indicted on the same score in similar studies in Finland, Hawaii, and in Framingham, Massachusetts.

The finger is also pointed at overuse of alcohol as a generally recognized risk factor in men by Philip B. Gorelick, of Chicago's Michael Reese Hospital. Gorelick is optimistic that many strokes will be preventable simply because heavy drinking is a reversible risk factor.[5]

To date, unfortunately, similar studies have *not* been

made in women exclusively, even though 87 women were included in the Birmingham survey. As a result, we can make no projections for conclusive answers about the effects of drinking in women.

Nonetheless, researchers for the English study do believe that heavy alcohol intake induces stroke by changing blood clotting components or by altering the pressure of blood flow.

Temperature Can Make the Difference

For the sake of a sound body and mind, there are some little-known facts about alcohol that everyone should know. A rise in body temperature, for example, increases alcohol's potency, and a fall in body temperature decreases its effects to a degree.

Experiments conducted at the Institute of Toxicology at the University of Southern California's School of Pharmacy indicate that alcohol impairs heat regulation in warm-blooded animals. This impairment causes body temperatures to fluctuate more in the direction of environmental temperature.[6]

"Usually, a warm-blooded animal holds its body temperature fairly constant," states Ronald L. Alkana, a professor of pharmacology. "With alcohol, a warm-blooded animal becomes more like a cold-blooded animal, changing body temperature with the ambient temperature."

Three things—alcohol, environmental temperature, and body temperature—can bring about a doubly charged effect, points out Alkana.

A usually safe intake of alcohol could be harmful or fatal in a hot environment—the tropics, for example. First, alcohol helps body temperature to rise, and, second, the higher body temperature heightens one's sensitivity to alcohol. A high intake under some conditions usually causes death due to respiratory failure.

At low body temperature, alcohol poses a different hazard: hypothermia. Body temperature can drop so low that heart and other organ functions are impaired and, again, death can result.

By necessity, these alcohol experiments have been limited to laboratory animals. Alkana does claim, however, that the findings may have important implications for human beings.

For instance, a soak in a hot tub might turn a nonlethal intake of alcohol into a lethal dose by significantly raising body temperature. Similarly, alcohol may pose fatal risks if consumed under extreme conditions—while a person is skiing on frigid slopes in Sun Valley or the Alps or is stranded in the relentless heat of the desert sun.

The Thief of Vitamin B-1

The intake of alcohol need not be high to cause complications. As a simple carbohydrate, alcohol requires vitamin B-1 (thiamine) for breaking it down to release energy. A diet of highly processed food furnishes little, if any, vitamin B-1.

White flour and white rice are examples of common foods that have been processed almost to death. The nutrition-rich germ and hull of the wheat have been milled away—the parts richest in thiamine. The same is true of rice. The polishing has been discarded, and the devitalized white rice remains. (Even so-called "enrichment" doesn't return all the needed nutrients to rice and other grains.)

How vital is B-1? Let's turn to an incident in the South Pacific and Oriental nations that occurred early in the twentieth century to find out. An acute thiamine deficiency caused an epidemic of beriberi. Numerous people suffered an inability to concentrate and remember, loss of energy, pain and paralysis of the limbs, edema (fluid accumulation in the tissues), weakened heart, and susceptibility to premature death.

The name *beriberi*, in fact, comes from the Philippine

term meaning "I can't, I can't." And no term could be more exact for describing the fatigue of those with beriberi. Truly, they can't do much of anything.

But why and how the beriberi? Let's turn to the early pioneer in vitamin research Christiaan Eijkman, living then in the Dutch East Indies. It was Eijkman who discovered that beriberi is caused by a deficiency of vitamin B–1 in widely consumed white rice. As a result, vast populations returned to eating unmilled rice and conquered what seemed to be an unconquerable disease.

Now alcohol brings a double whammy to the cells of body and brain. It contains no vitally needed vitamin B–1 for its proper conversion to energy, so the little provided by other foods is stolen to process it. Second, it blocks biochemical action by thiamin.

One of the most devastating conditions of chronic alcoholism is the Wernicke-Korsakoff syndrome, a nervous system disorder involving loss of coordination, rolling eyeballs, delirium, loss of memory, and mental impairment.

Unless sufficient thiamine is supplied, blood glucose can't be converted into energy, and a high level of lactic acid accumulates. Patients suffer acute confusion, disorientation, paralysis of eye muscles, heart failure, and probable death.

Why Not Add Vitamin B–1 to Alcohol?

Patients who suffer from Wernicke-Korsakoff syndrome usually eat voraciously after they stop drinking—but all the wrong things, sugar-rich foods with refined carbohydrates to compensate for the alcohol. Of course, in doing so they merely sustain the same problem they began with: an overload of carbohydrates without enough vitamin B–1 to translate into energy. And the final result? More lactic acid to shock the system.

Thus, in hospitals serving patients with acute cases of

alcoholism, medical staff should follow this simple, but potentially life-saving, procedure: administer thiamin intravenously or orally, before giving alcoholic patients food.

In fact, some decades ago, two biochemists came up with the idea of fortifying alcoholic beverages with vitamin B–1. And why not! They only wished to prevent conditions from mild vitamin B–1 deficiency to Wernicke-Korsakoff syndrome itself. They even published a paper on this proposal, showing that millions of dollars could be saved by wiping out alcohol-related diseases.[7]

Their proposal did make it as far as several committee meetings, but no further. And as far as I can determine, nothing more on the proposal has been done.

In the real world, it is impossible to induce everyone to stop drinking. But if you do drink, even in modest amounts, don't forget to eat whole grain foods, sunflower seeds, beans, peas, brown rice, and whole oats and take a vitamin B–1 or a B–complex supplement to assure that you metabolize your alcohol properly.

Tobacco and Russian Roulette

Tobacco is another one of the CATS all too difficult to give up. Now too it is fashionable to smoke fine and costly cigars. Despite the anticancer and emphysema warnings about smoking, people persist. Smoking though is like Russian roulette. Some people die young or live impaired lives because of tobacco, while others, the lucky ones, live through it without serious illness or an abbreviated life.

For most of us, however, tobacco is hazardous, even for nonsmokers exposed to secondhand smoke. For example, nearly 100 studies reveal that children of smokers are more inclined than those of nonsmokers to develop bronchitis, emphysema, and pneumonia. Several studies indicate that spouses of heavy smokers are two to three and one-half times more likely to develop lung cancer than spouses of nonsmokers.

Smoking is certainly one of the greatest enemies of thinking and remembering. And while nicotine serves as a mental stimulant like caffeine, it also depresses thyroid gland function. In the long run, smoking sabotages mind and body and is a life-shortener.

More specifically, a report in the *Journal of the American Medical Association* reveals that nicotine activates the adrenal glands and induces the secretion of more adrenalin.[8] At the same time, smoking constricts blood vessels. In fact, tobacco smoke from a single cigarette can narrow blood vessels for as much as 40 minutes, as demonstrated in a study by biochemist O. Pelletier.[9]

This phenomenon takes place in blood vessels througout the brain and body. Poor blood circulation is visible in premature wrinkling of face, neck, and hands of smokers, caused by insufficient oxygen as well as free radical action.

Aside from many cancer-causatives in tobacco, the smoke also gives off carbon monoxide. This action tends to displace some of the oxygen in red blood corpuscles, causing an even greater oxygen deficit for those who light up.

Nonetheless, there is abundant research to show that various nutrients can help to lessen the negative consequences of smoking and protect thinking and remembering in the process. An in-depth review of medical literature by nutrition editor-writer Harold J. Taub demonstrated that a daily supplement of between 5,000 to 10,000 International Units of vitamin A offers some protection to vulnerable mucus membranes of the throat and lungs.[10]

What foods and supplements are richest in vitamin A? Cod liver oil, beef liver, carrots, yams, red peppers, egg yolk, cantaloupe, apricots, broccoli, swordfish, whitefish, nectarines, pumpkin, cheese, halibut, soybeans, watermelon, and mackerel.

Vitally Important For Smokers

Vitamin E is another protector of smokers and of the vitamin A that protects them. A study by experts at four major universities found vitamin E to be a staunch guard against tobacco smoke and nitrogen oxide and ozone in areas beset by smog, another form of smoke we had better be wary of.

Let's turn now to Karen Owens, a San Diego area biochemist-nutritionist, who has studied many decades of vitamin E research. Karen has found that the average American ingests only about 7 I.U.s of vitamin E daily—far under the 800 I.U.s that serve as protectors and were found, over a three-year period, to be safe. Karen also advocates taking D–alpha tocopherol (the natural vitamin E), rather than the more reasonably priced D1–alpha tocopherol.[11]

In regard to vitamin C, a much quoted study reveals that one cigarette can remove as much as 25 milligrams of the vitamin from mind and body. Vitamin C has been shown to help guard against bladder cancer and a wide range of pollutants in tobacco smoke. It is also a champion fighter of free radicals caused by metabolism, smoking, other environmental pollutants, and stress. Vitamin C also helps restore vitamin E to free radical fighting fitness when it has been depleted.

Zinc can also come to the aid of all smokers, and those who endure secondhand smoke, everywhere. A daily intake of from 15 to 30 milligrams of zinc helps to keep the immune system strong to resist pollutants from smoking while also helping to prevent enlargement of the prostate gland. This is my finding with patients over the last 25 years.

Pure White and Innocent?

Refined sugar comes last but far from least in the listing of CATS. Sugar appears so innocent, pure and white, and offers a taste that's so enticing that we jokingly talk about being addicted to sugar. But sugar does as alcohol does. It's a simple carbohydrate with no inherent vitamin B–1 to help the body metabolize it. Sugar thus often depletes the little, existing vitamin B–1 we do possess and need to metabolize real food.

Refined sugar may even aid in developing high blood pressure. Experiments by Richard A. Ahrens, Ph.D., while in the University of Maryland's College of Human Ecology, show that an excessive intake of refined sugar can cause high blood pressure. By giving supplemental sugar to human beings and lab animals, Ahrens was able to raise their blood pressure at will. He believes that excessive sugar contributes to inordinate sodium retention that in turn, elevates blood pressure. This is enough to make Dr. Ahrens put white sugar on his blacklist.[12]

Another response that refined sugar—any refined carbohydrate, as a matter of fact—can cause is hypoglycemia, low blood sugar. I mention this here because hypoglycemia has a definite bearing on how well the mind works.

For a moment though, let's take a close look at how low blood sugar can happen. Say that you eat a gooey sweet roll or a candy bar. You get a brief high. Sugar quickly enters your bloodstream. Your pancreas then secretes insulin to remove glucose from your blood and escort it into your cells.

In this circumstance, however, the amount of sugar causes the pancreas to overreact, secreting so much insulin that the sugar is removed too rapidly from the blood, creating a glucose deficit. As a result, your energy sinks lower than before and, with it, your morale and ability to think well.

The Revealing Gyland Survey

In a survey of 600 hypoglycemic patients, Stephen Gyland, M.D., of Jacksonville, Florida, found that there are approximately 40 symptoms of hypoglycemia. Dr. Gyland also rated them according to how many of his patients had each particular symptom.[13]

In a phone interview, Dr. Gyland revealed that inability to think efficiently, mental confusion, poor coordination, and forgetfulness were prominent on his list. Exhaustion, the symptom near the head of the list, is another obvious factor that discourages problem-solving.

Gyland also lists nervousness, irritability, exhaustion, faintness, depression, dizziness, drowsiness, headaches, digestive disorders, forgetfulness, and inability to sleep as among the most serious symptoms.

If a glucose tolerance test establishes that you are hypoglycemic, what can you do to correct it? Here I advise prevention: cut out or cut down on simple carbohydrates such as refined sugar—in candy, cookies, cake, and other pastries. Canned fruits are also "no-no's" because of their high sugar content. Temporarily, I also rule out fruit and vegetables that are high in carbohydrates. Unfortunately, bananas, sweet cherries, grape juice, prunes and prune juice, sweet potatoes, kidney, lima and navy beans, corn, and hominy all have a 20 percent carbohydrate content.

Lowest carbohydrate content fruits and vegetables—in the 7 percent category—are grapefruit, lemons, strawberries, watermelon, and avocados, carrots, cauliflower, okra, onions, olives, peppers, pumpkin, and radishes.

USABLE FOODS	AVOIDABLE FOODS
Beef, lamb, poultry	Sugar (all types)
Fish	Candies, cake, pastries, pies, and raisins
Cheese, milk, yogurt, raisins, kefir	Macaroni, spaghetti, white rice
Vegetables (excluding those high in carbohydrate content)	Sweetened soft drinks without caffeine
Whole grain cereal and bread	Alcohol
Soybeans and their products	Coffee
Nuts (preferably unsalted)	Processed cereals
Eggs (unless you are hypocholesterolemic)	
Butter (unless you are hypocholesterolemic)	
Low carbohydrate fruits	

The most healthful way to consume foods containing sugar and starches (carbohydrates) is to eat foods low on the Glycemic Index Scale.

The Glycemic Index is the scientific measurement of how high an insulin response we get after eating a certain food. It's a hair-trigger response and the repercussion physiologically could cause low blood sugar.

By eating low Glycemic Index food and taking nutritional supplements—the multivitamin/mineral and essential fatty acids—you will not only reduce your incidence of hypoglycemia but lose weight rapidly as well. Insulin stores fat in body cells.

Low Glycemic Index foods are eggs, meat, fish, milk and plain yogurt, beans and peas, peaches, plums, pure fructose (fruit sugar), soybeans, peanuts and green vegetables. With the exception of peanuts, these foods will trigger the lowest insulin response. (We are aware of the pros and cons of milk, as well as the politics of it.)

Moderate Glycemic Index foods—which may be eaten in moderation—are nuts, bran cereal, brown rice, whole grain bread, grapes, sweet potatoes, whole grain wheat, whole grain flour pasta, pears, orange juice, apple juice, pineapple juice, oranges, apples, and oatmeal.

High Glycemic Index foods—which you should avoid whenever possible—include white bread, white potatoes, parsnips, carrots, corn, cornflakes, refined sugar, millet, beets, bananas, white rice, refined flour pasta, raisins, soda crackers, candy, cookies, cakes, and other pastries. (Crackers, candy, cookies, cake and other pastries also contain trans fats and oxidized cholesterol, enemies of the arteries and heart.)

One of my favorite diet counteractors to low blood sugar is five or six small meals daily to maintain blood sugar above the danger levels, using eatable foods for those who have hypoglycemia.

So much for coffee, alcohol, tobacco and sugar, the CATS that Dr. Braly warned about. Use them in moderation—or eliminate them, if you can. This way you can protect that investment between your ears and think and remember efficiently through the years.

CHAPTER 7

Heavy Metals and Your Brain

A frightening statistic about the amount of lead in the average person's body, cited in the first chapter, is on the verge of becoming alarming!

The National Academy of Sciences states that the average blood levels of lead in Americans today are from 500 to 1,000 times greater than those in bones of prehistoric individuals.

This means that with so much lead in the body, a great deal ends up in the brain and can reduce your I.Q. and your ability to think, make motor control difficult, cause a loss of balance, and invite other mental and physical problems. So states Dr. Hassan A.N. El-Fawal, at New York University's Institute of Environmental Medicine. Lead can also elevate blood pressure.[1]

The blood–brain barrier, a biological sievelike apparatus surrounding the brain, is supposed to protect us, and does a great deal of the time. But lead is another story, the lead molecule being small enough to slip on through to do its damage freely.

Inasmuch as more than two decades have passed since leaded gasoline has been discontinued, people wonder where lead originates. Exhaust from millions of cars worldwide for many years didn't just disappear. Lead is still in the air we breathe, in the water we drink, and in the food we eat.

Although lead-based paints were also banned many years ago, they still exist on the walls of many old homes, apartments, and tenements. As they oxidize, they become dust that we breathe in. Industrial plants that exhale lead and other contaminants from their smokestacks are still in use as well. Then there's the sewage sludge we use for fertilizer that passes lead on to vegetables and fruit—and finally to us.

Tobacco smoke also contains lead. And what about the lead-soldered water pipes and canned food containers, lead-glazed ceramics and earthenware, insect killers sprayed on fruit trees and tobacco—they also contain the poison arsenic—and toothpaste tubes. An unsuspected source of lead is hair-coloring products. In fact, lead is as much around us as the amounts we willingly or unwillingly take into us.

Damage That Lead Can Do

Sellers of gasoline were able to get the lead out. Now how do we get the lead out of our anatomy?

Before answering that question though, let's take a closer look at what lead does to us, first as children where it is most devastating. Perhaps the world's foremost authority on this subject is Dr. Herbert L. Needleman, a psychiatrist at the University of Pittsburgh School of Medicine, a former member of the Harvard Medical School faculty.

Perhaps Dr. Needleman's most significant study involves boys ages 7 to 11 showing high lead concentrations in their bones. His research revealed that these boys have problems paying attention (making it difficult to take in new information) and thinking, have lower-than-normal I.Q.s and show aggressive behavior and delinquency.

In sharp contrast, boys in matched age and background

groups with low to moderate concentrations of lead in their bones exhibit none or far fewer of these traits and tendencies.

"These data argue that environmental lead exposure, a preventable occurrence, should be included when considering the many factors contributing to delinquent behavior," the investigator told a *Science News* reporter.[2]

Dr. Needleman and associates took into account the major variables—for instance, differences in mothers' schooling, I.Q.s and occupations—in comparing the boys with high and low lead bone concentrations. After comparing for two-parent homes and adequate child-rearing practices, results remained unchanged.

This study of 212 Pittsburgh public school boys confirms findings of earlier, smaller scale research projects.

Additional studies by Terrie E. Moffitt, a psychologist at the University of Wisconsin–Madison, show similar results: attention deficit disorder, low intelligence, and aggressive behavior of boys with a heavy lead burden—possible predictors of delinquency, violent crime, alcoholism, and domestic abuse.

"Links between such measures and lead exposure warrant careful attention," Moffitt told *Science News*.

How to Banish Your Load of Lead

A study by biochemist Rhoda Papaioannou and associates at the Brain Bio Center in Princeton, New Jersey, reveals an effective way of dealing with such lead loads and even lead poisoning. They studied 22 workers in a battery factory where the air was heavy with lead and the absentee rate due to lead poisoning was super-high.[3]

The Brain Bio researchers administered 2000 milligrams of vitamin C and 60 milligrams of zinc daily to the lead-poisoned workers.

Prior to going on this regimen, the workers were tested for blood levels of lead and also after 6, 12, and 24 week intervals. Results were promising after 24 weeks. Blood levels of lead had dropped by 26 percent, and workers showed fewer symptoms of lead poisoning.

Rhoda Papaioannou reported the following: "These changes were striking in view of the fact that they were achieved while the workers were on the job and constantly exposed to high levels of lead."

The researchers theorized that the vitamin C and zinc prevented absorption of more lead from the digestive tract and found a way of removing it from the blood.

Projecting their findings to the general public, the researchers felt that this protocol might protect our body and mind from the devastating assault from lead until—or if—the environment is cleaned up.

For more than a century, chemists have known that pectin, that gelatinous substance used to make jellies congeal, could also help to prevent lead poisoning. When pectin, derived from sunflower seeds, apples or grapefruit, meets our digestive juices, it is transformed to galacturonic acid that converts lead—also other heavy metals—into insoluble metal salts that can't be absorbed and, therefore, are thrown off in body wastes. You can find pectin products in many of the health food stores in cities everywhere.

Chelation Can Do the Trick

Chelation is a third effective way of ridding the body of lead. EDTA, the chelation solution, binds with lead and forcibly ejects it from the body.

Chelation is not a Johnny-Come-Lately therapy with no history of success either. During World War II, medical researchers discovered that EDTA could help in removing lead from the human system. This was especially important for workers in battery factories and individuals painting warships with lead-based paints who were sooner or later disabled with lead poisoning.

Intravenous dripping of the synthetic protein EDTA into the arteries of these individuals removed the lead and restored them to good health. Actually, it did even more. Researchers noticed that it also reduced the symptoms of heart disease in many patients, permitting an easier flow of blood to and from the heart and the brain.

Despite the fact that there have been hundreds of thousands of successful chelations, the medical establishment still does not recognize this safe and effective therapy. Chelation therapy has even been found helpful in removing another one of the deadliest poisons in the human body: cadmium.

This killer pollutant, known to cause birth defects, decrease mental ability, and promote high blood pressure and heart ailments is widely used to make pigments, plastics, and stabilizers for motor oil, and to refine zinc. Little-recognized sources of cadmium are tobacco and tobacco smoke and our streets and highways.

Fungicides sprayed on growing tobacco can also contain cadmium, which invades tobacco leaves, and ends up in inhaled smoke in lungs, blood, body, and brain cells. Cadmium is also leached from water pipes by soft water.

Used in the hardening of rubber tires, cadmium dust is deposited on streets, freeways, and highways, where we breathe it in. Cadmium is a stubborn resident in our body and brain cells, where it accumulates over the years. There it can cause iron deficiency anemia, through which it short-changes us of hemoglobin that carries oxygen to the brain and slows our thinking and remembering. It can cause high blood pressure, emphysema, and kidney ailments.

Zinc Can Help the Cause

In the book *Toxic Metal Syndrome,* Richard Casdorph, M.D., and Morton Walker, M.D., write that "In humans, the urine of hypertensive patients contains up to 40 percent more cadmium than does the urine of normotensive (normal) persons."[4]

Abundant research indicates that a sufficient intake of zinc can prevent cadmium from finding receptor sites in cells. Drs. Casdorph and Walker suggest that taking 15 milligrams of zinc with breakfast and another 15 mg with dinner is a good way to prevent cadmium toxicity.

Chelation therapy is also successful in removing cadmium from body and brain fluids, as demonstrated by before and after hair analysis.

The Environmental Protection Agency (EPA) is constantly setting acceptable toxicity levels of harmful pollutants for children and adults. And authorities in the field are constantly finding them far too high.

This finding is borne out by an in-depth study by Mike Marlowe, chairman of the Department of Language, Reading and Exceptionalities at Appalachian State University, and Charles Moon, chairman of the Department of Education at Heidelberg College in Tiffin, Ohio.[5]

Their findings are based on lead, cadmium, and mercury measurements of 59 children drawn from a general school population.

"A continuing reexamination of metal exposure (to lead, cadmium and mercury) and metal-metal interactions (lead and cadmium or cadmium and mercury, for example) previously thought harmless and routinely experienced in the environment, may be associated with intellectual decrease or loss," states Marlowe.

Citing numerous research reports, Marlowe indicates that children who survive metal poisoning are at risk for mental retardation via damage done to their central nervous systems.

Even children with a moderate increase in body toxic metals—although clinically without symptoms—may also be subject to impaired mental development but is somewhat more difficult to define.

We do know this: a definite relationship exists between low to moderate levels of metals, until recently thought to be harmless, with psychological deficits and central nervous system dysfunctions. Even interactions of low concentrations of metals have a negative synergistic association with psychologic performance.

Mercury: The Silent Enemy

Mercury, the silvery fluid found in thermometers, is a potent mind and body poison. Remember the phrase "mad as a hatter?" In past centuries, hat makers processed their materials with mercury and soon developed brain damage, intensified by bizarre conduct, mental fuzziness, and memory loss.

In addition mercury's toxicity can cause chest pain, chills, weakness, fever, kidney damage, loose teeth, irritability, nervousness, and loss of sex drive.

Even a low level of mercury toxicity can contribute to brain damage, kidney dysfunction, injury to the liver as well as to the pancreas and bone marrow. (The bone marrow is the place where blood cells are made.) Mercury can severely aggravate high blood pressure and diabetes.

Mercury is a pernicious body and mind poison. It attacks protein by changing its structure and rendering it physiologically useless. This can be devastating when you consider that our trillions of cells are made of protein and that antibodies—key parts of our immune system—enzymes, hemoglobin and hormones are proteins.

Aside from the natural mercury in the earth's crust that is then released into streams, lakes and oceans, the soil and air, there are many more manmade sources.

Do You Have a Mouth Full of Mercury?

There has been an ongoing war among experts regarding amalgam fillings in our teeth, which contain as much as 40 percent mercury. Dentists must follow strict regulations in storing, handling, using, and disposing of this highly toxic metal.

Consider this: The EPA designates scrap amalgam fillings as hazardous waste. The Occupational Safety and Health Adminstration (OSHA) has a special handling procedure for scrap amalgam that is mandatory to follow. If mercury-laden fillings are highly toxic outside the mouth, they are certainly toxic when they're in our teeth.

Hal Huggins, D.D.S., of Colorado Springs, Colorado, has taken a beating professionally—even losing his license to practice—because he dared to oppose the continued use of amalgam fillings for teeth. He cited the cases of 200 patients who suffered from a vast assortment of medical disorders associated with mercury-laden fillings and their recovery when these fillings were replaced by harmless nonmetallic materials.[6]

The Eggleston Experiment

Based on medical literature that made mercury fillings suspect, David W. Eggleston, D.D.S., a clinical professor of the Department of Restorative Dentistry at the University of Southern California, launched his own investigation of the issue.

In his private practice in Newport Beach, California, he enlisted test subjects who, for research purposes, agreed to have all of their amalgam fillings removed and, then, replaced with nonmetallic fillings.

Jim Scheer, my collaborator, took part in Dr. Eggleston's preliminary study, offering blood samples for analysis before and after removal of his amalgam fillings.

When the experiment ended, the number of Jim's T–

lymphocyte cells in ratio to total lymphocyte cells, rose by more than 30 percent, showing an appreciable strengthening of his immune system function.

Let's look at this finding in a little more depth. White blood cells called lymphocytes are produced in the lymph glands. Those that pass through the thymus gland, the immune system's master gland, are changed into T–lymphocytes. As we add years, the thymus gland shrinks, and its hormone production is reduced.

This reduction is thought to be a major reason that so many cancers occur later in life and also why automimmune disorders are so prevalent at this time. In autoimmunity our defender cells attack the body they are supposed to defend. It makes good sense, therefore, to give the immune system all the help it can get.

Another of Dr. Eggleston's studies of the amalgam issue revealed the results of autopsy research: There is far more mercury in the brain tissue of bodies with mercury-laden amalgam fillings than in others.[7]

Mercury's 100-Year War On Us

Late in the 1970s, Willem H. Khoe, M.D., who practices preventive medicine in Las Vegas, Nevada, studied medical journal publications on the issue of amalgam fillings for the previous 100 years and found that most of the papers revealed mercury fillings as *harmful* to our health.

There is some evidence that alpha lipoic acid, a powerful antioxidant, is effective in removing mercury from the human system. Chelation therapy, too, has been successful in removing mercury, as well as other biochemical debris that narrows arteries and sometimes blocks them.

CHAPTER 8

Stress: The Mind-Killer

Several years ago, the negative influence of stress was dramatically demonstrated by Alan C. Yeung, M.D., a cardiologist at Harvard Medical School, and associates.[1]

The Yeung team studied 26 volunteers—women and men—who had chest pains symptomatic of coronary artery disease. By means of angiography, a special X-ray technique, they viewed the subjects' three coronary arteries, the main blood vessels to the heart.

Then they classified the interior of these arteries as "relatively smooth," "irregular" (with a small amount of plaque), or "stenosed" (almost clogged with plaque).

Next they subjected the volunteers to mental stress and, again, studied their coronary arteries. What they saw was amazing. Stress had caused the arteries with the most atherosclerotic plaque to narrow even more, reducing blood flow to the heart. Potentially, this narrowing could have led to a heart attack.

During the test, the most stenosed (plaque-filled) arteries constricted by 24 percent. Arteries with little plaque constricted by 9 percent. Yet, there was no perceptible constriction in the smooth and healthy arteries.

They checked their results by another method: volume of blood flow. Flow decreased by 27 percent in both the extremely and mildly clogged arteries. In sharp contrast, it *increased* by 10 percent in the smooth arteries.

Why? The smooth lining of healthy arteries can expand more and permit the flow of more blood. The researchers theorize that when the hormone epinephrine sends out the message for these vessels to constrict, the smooth lining of healthy blood vessels secretes a substance called endothelium-derived relaxing factor (EDRF).

"Healthy vessels secrete ERDF to balance the constricting effect of epinephrine," Yeung told the American Heart Association's 64th session. "But if you have unhealthy vessels, that balancing act is gone."

Such artery constriction—even spasms—takes place under stressful conditions in any part of the body or brain. Many medical doctors who perform chelation treatments find that the lining of the carotid artery—the main artery that supplies blood to the brain—is frequently filled with plaque. Under stressful conditions, it then limits blood flow, reducing oxygen and glucose entering the brain.

A Reasonable Alternative

One natural solution here is to take large doses of vitamin C daily. This proposal is based on my 30 years of study and use of vitamin C and its protective influences in keeping my patients' arteries smooth and their hearts beating regularly and efficiently.

Some years ago, Jim Scheer and I attended the First World Congress on vitamin C in Palm Springs, California. We were fortunate to spend some private time with up-in-years, white-haired, Nobel prize winner Albert Szent-Gyorgyi, M.D., the conference's primary speaker, who, in 1928, discovered vitamin C.

Dr. Szent-Gyorgyi told us that diseases of the artery—and the heart—are essentially a form of scurvy, what the *New World Dictionary of the American Language* defines as "a disease resulting from a deficiency of vitamin C in the body, characterized by weakness, anemia, spongy gums and bleeding from the mucus membranes."

At the time, what Dr. Szent-Gyorgyi said appeared to be too sweeping a generality, even from someone who knew more about vitamin C—and, probably, scurvy—than anyone else in the world.

Later, we came across corroborating research by Dr. Anthony Verlangieri, then at Rutgers University. In experiments with rabbits, Dr. Verlangieri discovered that a diet deficient in vitamin C caused a loss of chemical compounds in the once smooth artery linings (the intima), creating irregularities, soon filled by plaques of cholesterol, fats, ceroids, and calcium. A diet high in vitamin C prevented this from happening. The intima remained smooth.[2]

More than 22 years of experiments by Dr. M.L. Riccitelli, of the Yale School of Medicine, validated the Verlangieri findings.[3]

Dr. Riccitelli reported on a study of vitamin C-deprived guinea pigs that showed irregularities of the intima almost identical to those of human beings with atherosclerosis. (Guinea pigs are one of the few animals that can't synthesize vitamin C.) The revealing aspect of this experiment was that the sick arteries of the guinea pigs were completely healed with prolonged vitamin C therapy.

Also reported by Dr. Riccitelli was that other researchers, 20 years before his own experiments, had shown that vitamin C reduces cholesterol levels and blocks the buildup of cholesterol, fats, and calcium on artery walls.

Unfortunately though, "Very little has been reported in the literature regarding the effects of vitamin C in the etiology of atherosclerosis," he wrote.

The reason for this lack is clear: Orthodox researchers

were so busy trying to deal with the symptom—reducing cholesterol and LDL cholesterol, the worst kind—that the fundamentals escaped them.

Scurvy Revealed in the Arteries

Several other investigators after Dr. Riccitelli, discovered that animals deprived of vitamin C developed atherosclerotic lesions—what Dr. Albert Szent-Gyorgyi had called a sign of scurvy—and were cured by vitamin C treatments over a long period.

Sadly, like certain types of monkeys, the guinea pig, the red-whiskered bulbul (a bird), and the fruit-eating Indian bat, we human beings lack a certain enzyme in our livers, preventing us from making vitamin C from glucose. This means we have to take in this vitamin from the outside.

Certainly, our needs for it vary. But if we don't satisfy our requirements, we may develop a number of diseases, including hardening of the arteries.

One of the final studies by the late Dr. Linus Pauling, two-time Nobel Laureate, bears out the Szent-Gyorgyi theory. It was conducted with Matthias Rath, M.D., then director of Cardiovascular Research at the Linus Pauling Institute of Science and Medicine in Palo Alto, California.

Actually, the study also confirms, elaborates, and explains the discoveries of Drs. Verlangieri and Riccitelli. As Dr. Pauling wrote:

> Heart disease is an epidemic disease. Most epidemic diseases are caused by a single factor: an insuffient intake of vitamin C that leads to destabilization of the walls of blood vessels.
>
> After our ancestors had lost the ability to manufacture vitamin C in their bodies, the blood vessel system became the most vulnerable site of the human body. . . . Millions of our ancestors died of scurvy and blood loss.

In several papers, Dr. Rath validates the Pauling and Szent-Gyorgyi position that deteriorating arteries are a form of scurvy. With modern viewing technology such as ultrafast computed tomography, calcified deposits of cholesterol and other fats are clearly visible.

How Vitamin C Does It

An amazing statistic from Dr. Rath will shock you into attention. His studies of animals and human beings reveal atherosclerosis to be such an aggressive disease that it can worsen by an annual average of 44 percent! Imagine that!

However, he claims that it can be stopped with ample vitamin C. In many cases, a year's therapy with vitamin C demonstrated that artery-clogging deposits disappear.

In one of his publications issued by the Linus Pauling Heart Foundation, "Solution to the Puzzle of Human Cardiovascular Disease," Dr. Rath writes:

"If you don't get enough vitamin C, your body cannot produce adequate collagen, and collagen is the substance that gives your cardiovascular system structural integrity. Low vitamin C intake over many years leads to chronic instability of the vessel walls."[4]

Dr. Rath likens collagen to the steel girders that give a skyscraper structural integrity. Taking too little vitamin C shuts off collagen production, and the interior of the blood vessels and arteries loses its structural integrity.

With the weakening of the blood vessels, tiny lesions (injuries) develop in the blood vessel interior, which then loses elasticity. The body compensates by sending cholesterol and fatty material to patch the damage.[5]

Actually, the body overcompensates, says Dr. Rath. "It overshoots the repair mechanism. Arterial deposits are nothing more than nature's 'plaster cast' against the weakness of blood vessel walls."

Current belief holds that low density lipoprotein (LDL,

considered the bad form of cholesterol) is a villain of the cardiovascular scenario. For Drs. Rath and Pauling, however, lipoprotein(a), known by the acronym Lp(a), is the main ingredient in deposits on the interior of blood vessels, not LDL.

In fact, Lp(a) is made from LDL and a substance called apo(a) formed in the liver. Deterioration of arteries and consequent patching is mainly a degenerative disease caused by "a deficiency of vitamin C."

An Artery Protection Plan That Works

These findings—from Dr. Szent-Gyorgyi to Drs. Rath and Pauling—make me, in my medical practice, emphasize sufficient vitamin C to prevent scurvy of the arteries to the heart, throughout the body and in the mind.

I recommend that my patients take at least 500 milligrams of vitamin C after each meal, preferably in crystalline or capsule form, because this is more easily digested and absorbed than in pill form. Vitamin C rarely remains in the human system for more than eight hours. If you take it three times daily, there's always some vitamin C working in your system.

Special care must be taken storing crystalline vitamin C to retain its strength. The container must be tightly sealed and kept in a cool dark place. Capsules containing crystalline vitamin C are not quite as temperamental and subject to degeneration by oxygen and light.

My patients who show signs of atherosclerosis have seen their condition corrected within a year or more by this regimen. It is satisfying to know that their blood flow is powerful and reaches all areas of body and mind.

So far, we've dealt with the effects of stress on arteries. Now let's look at stress itself, how to avoid it, and, also, how to cope with it before it damages our arteries.

How to Conserve Your Adrenal Glands

In the real world, from time to time, we are exposed to stressors—mental, emotional and physical—that activate the two tiny, yellow adrenal glands that fit like caps on top of the kidneys. Short, intermittent stressors help to keep the adrenal glands working properly.

Repeated long-enduring stressors or single, severe ones, like the loss of a loved one, do just the opposite—they deplete your hard-earned adrenal hormones. It's much like keeping your car's starter grinding away when the ignition refuses to fire, and you drain your storage battery. In this way, over the years, it is possible to wear out the adrenal glands—and you may not be able to recharge them. Take my advice. Use preventive measures *now!*

Some stressors are obvious and easy to detect. Others—if not most—are subtle and not easily detectable, especially those that originate in emotional conflict.

Here is a list of telltale signs and symptoms that help me to alert my patients that they are being stressed. If you have seven or more of the following, there's a good chance you may be overstressed.

1. Cold extremities—hands and feet—even if your thyroid gland is working normally on its own or helped by natural thyroid gland supplementation
2. Gritting teeth (a condition called "bruxism" in medicalese)
3. Eyestrain (tightness of the eyes and frequent nervous blinking)
4. Many headaches or a sustained one (symptomatic of many medical conditions)
5. Hypertension (high blood pressure)
6. Hair-trigger irritability
7. Shallow or irregular breathing
8. Nervous jittering of knees while seated

9. Frequent tapping of fingers
10. Decrease or sharp increase of food intake
11. Decided loss of sense of humor
12. Loss of interest in sex
13. Inability to fall asleep or sustain sleep
14. Repeated oversleeping
15. Constant stomach upset
16. Worrying that makes thinking difficult
17. Decided increase in drinking
18. Decided increase in smoking
19. Excessive use of tranquilizers
20. Inability to relax
21. Feeling unable to face problems
22. Nonstop anxiety

Highest Stress Work

Another way to determine whether or not you are overstressed is to examine your occupation or profession. Is it threatened by layoffs due to computerization, mechanization, robotics, or other advanced technology? Are you under the gun to meet frequent and rigid deadlines? Is your work hazardous? Are you responsible for the job future or lives of others?

If even one or more of these fits your situation, you are likely to be job- or profession-stressed.

An international authority on occupational stress and associates conducted a study for the British *Sunday Times* to determine the most stressful occupations relative to incidence of alcoholism, heart attacks, heavy smoking, nervous breakdowns, job burnout and divorces.

The authority is Cary L. Cooper, Ph.D., professor of organizational psychology, Department of Management Sciences at the University of Manchester, England, Institute of Sciences and Technology. Following are the ratings of occupations in descending order from ten to one of the stress they generate. Dr. Cooper related them to Jim Scheer in a telephone interview[6]:

Stress: The Mind-Killer 111

Obviously each one of us differs in how we react to our work, and circumstances of each category of job or profession differs.

Miner	8.3
Police officer	7.7
Construction worker	7.5
Journalist	7.5
Commercial pilot	7.5
Prison officer	7.5
Advertising executive	7.3
Dentist	7.3
Actor	7.2
Politician	7.0
Doctor (medical)	6.8
Tax collector	6.8
Film producer	6.5
Nurse	6.5
Firefighter	6.3
Musician	6.3
Teacher	6.2
Personnel director	6.0
Social worker	6.0
Public relations officer	5.8
Manager	5.7
Sales clerk	5.7
Stockbroker	5.5
Bus driver	5.4
Psychologist	5.2
Publishing executive	5.0
Diplomat	4.8
Farmer	4.8
Soldier	4.7
Veterinarian	4.5
Civil servant	4.4
Accountant	4.3
Engineer	4.3

Real estate broker	4.3
Hair stylist	4.3
Secretary	4.3
Lawyer	4.3
Artist, designer	4.2
Architect	4.0
Optician	4.0
Planner (city, county, state)	4.0
Letter carrier	4.0
Statistician	4.0
Lab technician	3.8
Banker	3.7
Computer operator	3.7
Occupational therapist	3.7
Linguist	3.7
Clergy	3.5
Nursery school assistant	3.5
Astronomer	3.4
Museum worker	2.8
Librarian	2.0

Zero in on Your Stressors

Dr. Cooper suggests that you precisely identify your stressors, then try to deal with them—no matter what your work or profession is. In fact, there are five areas for zeroing in on occupational stress: (1) problems with the work itself; (2) problems with your role in the company or organization; (3) problems with your career; (4) problems with work relationships; and (5) problems with company or organizational structure or climate.

Relative to the job or profession, you may be stressed by one of the following as well:

1. Poor working conditions: high noise level, intense heat, accident hazards without enough protection, crowded quarters, or clutter.

Stress: The Mind-Killer

2. Physical danger, as in police work or fire protection (this stressor responds most readily to taking available training and using all equipment that makes the work safer).
3. Handling hazardous materials or confidential reports.
4. Overload of work: too much to do; inability to perform the job or assignment properly; or feeling incapable of delivering.
5. Rigid schedules and severe time pressure.

Other sources of stress come from the company or the organization itself, including: (1) not understanding your specific role; (2) doing work you dislike or things you think you shouldn't have to do; and (3) having and fearing responsibility for others.

A career itself supplies its own kinds of stressors: inability to win a promotion or higher wages or salary, or being overpromoted and feeling inadequate for the new work and fearful of losing the job or position.

Dr. Cooper reminds us that relationships can be sources of conflict or frustration and, therefore, stressors: negative relations with your boss, coworkers, or subordinates. You may also have problems in delegating work or handling your immediate responsibility.

Organizational structure, policy, or climate can be added sources of stress: being left out of the decision-making process, facing limited budgets that restrict goals and plans, and frustrations in dealing with office politics.

How to Cope With Your Stress

Once you have identified your stressor or stressors, Dr. Cooper advises you to take remedial action. You can make your boss aware of it (them) and enlist his or her cooperation in taking corrective action. This may take persistence carried on in a diplomatic manner.

Should you feel that your knowledge about the work is limited, study and fill in your areas of weakness. Doing so will help banish feelings of inferiority or job insecurity and reduce stress. Dr. Cooper suggests trying to take a more positive attitude toward your work. If that doesn't help, you might seek a transfer within the organization or company. If all else fails, you might try to find a new place to work before resigning from your present position.

Dr. Cooper has various stress-reducing measures that have helped his clients and students.

"Running, sauna, meditation and biofeedback all make positive contributions," he says. He continues:

> By meditation I mean finding a quiet place and detaching yourself from the world and its problems—quiet relaxation. These are useful techniques to help you cope with the causes of stress. However, remember first to deal with the basics, the underlying problems, because only by doing that will you get rid of the causes of stress.

Stressors come in all shapes, colors, and sizes—physical, emotional, or mental. Marathon running, cross-country skiing, handball, hockey, heavy lifting (as done by stevedores, sandhogs, or longshoremen) are typical physical stressors, along with exposure to extremes of cold or heat, exposure to radiation, involvement in a car accident, or reaction to any serious illness.

Some of the most severe emotional stressors are loss of a job, moving to a new community or job, serious illness in the family, or death of a spouse. Others are hatred, long-held grudges, anxiety, and fear, all of which impair gastrointestinal efficiency and cause poor digestion, absorption, and assimilation of food. These physical responses in turn, make fewer nutrients available to your body and deprive you of fuel needed for work, play, and coping with other stressors.

Mental stressors include having to learn a foreign language for practical use within several days, preparing for and taking an arduous exam for a professional license, or having to grapple with a problem that no one else has been able to solve.

How Stress Can Harm You

Once you realize the physical, mental, and emotional consequences of stressors, you will understand why certain organs of the body suffer and as they do so deprive the brain of its rightful supply of oxygen and nutrients.

Let's consider what extreme stress or long-enduring moderate stress can do. In "fight or flight" situations, you need every ounce of energy to supply the large muscles for instant, strenuous action.

Various hormones in the blood trigger the adrenal glands, and a chemical emergency procedure breaks loose. The adrenal glands' cortex (outer layer) and the medulla (center) release hormones. Those released by the adrenal cortex sound the alarm. Blood pressure rises dramatically for quicker delivery of energy fuel. Blood sugar level soars to supply fuel for the emergency. Digestion stops to conserve energy for the crisis. Proteins from the thymus and lymph glands are converted to sugar for instant energy. The liver is alerted to convert glycogen (a form of stored sugar) into glucose.

Minerals are drawn out of the bones. Fat is marshalled from storage areas. Heartbeat and breathing are accelerated. Rapidly recruited biochemical raw materials are speeded to the front to repair critical areas of tissue.

There is no promissory note to pay back raw materials borrowed under the emergency. If they are not repaid, certain areas and organs of the body—and the brain, too—will suffer. If the diet is substantial and well supplied with the right supplements, borrowed materials are slowly paid back in the postemergency period. And there's no harm done.

What's Going on Inside

Continued stress, however, will keep the body in the emergency mode and not in a position to pay back borrowed biochemical materials. Coupled with a deficient diet, stress drives the body and mind into exhaustion. Tissue repairs can't be made, and serious illness results with a possibility of death.

Incessant stress causes life-supporting protein to be drawn out of the glandular first lines of defense: the thymus (master gland of the immune system), the lymph glands (also a part of this defense network), and the adrenal glands. Continued heavy stress causes the thymus and lymph glands to shrivel and atrophy.

And the beat goes on. As the desperate need for protein continues, the body steals it from wherever it can: blood plasma, kidneys, liver, and stomach.

Stomach lesions result from protein being cannibalized from the stomach walls. Ulcerative colitis can be caused by protein drawn from the intestinal lining. Similar self-destruction is taking place in the bones, with the removal of calcium and other critical minerals.

Prodigious amounts of protein are used in one day of super-stress: the protein supplied by four quarts of milk, as measured by the tremendous loss of nitrogen in the urine. It has been demonstrated in various studies that when high amounts of protein are supplied to meet the body's inordinate needs, the inner destruction is stopped.

For highly stressed individuals, an extra supply of vitamin A is essential for recovery, to keep the adrenal glands from swelling and then from overproducing cortisone that can destroy protection-giving lymph cells and shrink the thymus gland, weakening the immune system or, more dangerous yet, shutting it down.

Vitamins A and B–5 to the Rescue

Dr. Eli Seifter and associates at Albert Einstein Medical College in New York City demonstrated the protective effect of extra vitamin A in stress.[7]

Placing mice in a partial cast to prevent their normal movement, while not harming them, these researchers later examined the animals and found much enlarged adrenal glands and a shrunken thymus. After the mice were released, supplementary vitamin A restored the adrenal glands and the thymus to normal.

A deficiency of pantothenic acid (vitamin B–5) in a stressful situation causes the adrenal glands to shrivel and fill up with dead cellular debris and blood. This shortage of a critically needed vitamin limits the glands from producing their protective hormones. Stress and low intake of pantothenic acid can bring on physical complications and compound the effects of additional stress.

Pantothenic acid is an enabler. It helps cholesterol to be converted into adrenal, pituitary gland, and sex hormones. A minor deficiency in this vitamin reduces the amount of these hormones secreted. If the deficiency of pantothenic acid has not been long and severe, a high intake of this vitamin can again start the biochemical factory producing these hormones overnight.

Best food and supplement sources of pantothenic acid are royal jelly, brewer's and torula yeast, whole brown rice, sunflower seeds, corn, lentils, egg yolk, peas, alfalfa, whole wheat, whole rye, eggs, bee pollen, and wheat germ.

As with pantothenic acid, stress bleeds the system of vitamin C. A serious lack of vitamin C can cause adrenal glands to hemorrhage and sharply reduce hormone production.

It's Not the Stress—It's Your Response To It

In *Who Gets Sick,* a wonderful look at coping with stress, Blair Justice, Ph.D., offers dozens of examples to show that it is not the stressor that undermines us, but our attitude toward that stressor.[8]

Inasmuch as people don't avoid stress or learn to cope with it, they pay the penalty with tranquilizers, alcohol, exercise, or—later—a triple bypass. But the new evidence is that stress is not the problem. It is our response to it that largely determines health or sickness.

A group of behavioral scientists at the University of Chicago, led by psychologists Suzanne Kobasa and Salvatore Maddi, interviewed 200 executives of Illinois Bell Telephone Company, who had experienced the horrendous stress of insecurity during the AT&T divestiture, writes Dr. Justice.

One hundred of the officers and managers reported many symptoms of illness. The other hundred had few signs of llness. Why the difference? Dr. Kobasa and associates discovered that the excutives who stayed healthy had a different way of dealing with stressful events from the others.

The healthy managers attached no "good" or "bad" labels to the suspense or anxiety attached to changes. They considered them an inevitable part of life and a chance for growth and new experiences, not a threat to security. Their optimism gave them a sense of control. It was just the opposite for the other 100.

Best Ways to Beat Stress

"Those who stay healthy under stress, Kobasa found, have, in addition to a sense of control and challenge, a commitment to life," writes Dr. Justice. "They are deeply involved in their work and families, and their commitment gives them a sense of meaning, direction and excitement. They have acquired 'hardy' personalities, which help to protect them from illness."

Remember: It is our response to stress that's more important than the stress itself. And now, there is definite evidence that—in those who are not hardy personalities or respond poorly to problems—high levels of stress can do direct damage to the brain.

In an earlier chapter, we mentioned disastrous consequences of stress in terms of glucose (blood sugar). If high level stress persists, glucose is directed away from the brain in the hippocampus area to the muscles. Deprived of their food for too long a time, brain cells can die.

Here's another aspect to consider: the consequences of oxygen deprivation. Under stress, people become shallow breathers. When the stress continues unabated, the oxygen supply is constantly subnormal and may even be reduced to a dangerous level.

In their book *Psychochemistry,* Paul Gillette, Ph.D., and Marie Hornbeck describe such a scenario.[9] Student volunteers took part in an experiment in which the oxygen supply was slowly and progressively reduced. Mental performance, as measured by various psychological tests, steadily declined.

A study along the same lines some years ago by psychiatrist Ebbe Curtis Hoff, of the Medical College of Virginia, was most revealing, too. For *just three hours,* twenty-six students were exposed to air with only a 13 percent oxygen content, rather than normal air at sea level with about 20 percent oxygen.

All had difficulty concentrating, and their perception time was slowed. They also suffered headaches, dizziness, yawning, pains in joints, tingling fingers and toes, vague anxiety, moderate depression, reduced creativity, and difficulty in remembering.

There's more about memory in the chapter coming up: how to develop it, how to use it, and how to preserve it.

drinks, cocoa, chocolate or chocolate milk deplete the body's meager supply of vitamin B−1. So do high intakes of alcohol, refined sugar and flour, or of raw fish. (A fondness for frequently eaten sushi helped weaken the memory of one of my student patients.)

Several experiments with rats also demonstrate with impact that vitamin B−1 deficiency can undermine the memory.[2] In one experiment, rats trained to find their way through a maze were divided into two groups. The first group was given a nutritionally complete diet. The other group was fed rations that lacked vitamin B−1.

Three weeks later, the rats got their memory test. The group on the complete diet raced through the maze in an average time of 22 seconds flat. The vitamin B−1 deficient animals finally bumbled their way through in an average 55 seconds—about two and one-half times longer.

Later, when the deprived rats were brought up to speed with thiamin, they made a dramatic recovery in memory and solved the maze in record time.

A Study From Adelle Davis

Some years ago, the late Adelle Davis told Jim Scheer about "a fascinating experiment in memory revival with vitamin B−1" that she had observed.[3]

Patients at a Philadelphia hospital on diets low in vitamin B−1 were tested for memory and ability to think clearly and quickly. Results were subnormal compared with controls whose diets were adequate in vitamin B−1.

Then vitamin B−1 was injected into them.

"The change was incredible," Adelle Davis stated. "Their memory for recent and past events surprised even the researchers. Also, their ability to think clearly and quickly increased remarkably."

Why the change? Vitamin B−1 is essential for glucose to be converted into energy. Unless sufficient thiamine is present, toxic pyruvic and lactic acids accumulate in brain cells, reducing mental ability.

A vitamin B–1 deficiency also has greater ramifications relative to other body and brain nutrients. Too little vitamin B–1 lowers energy so that stomach muscle contractions weaken, decreasing their ability to secrete hydrochloric acid and digestive enzymes. As a result, digested food cannot properly contact absorbing surfaces in order to enter the bloodstream.

There's even more to the story. Insufficient hydrochloric acid makes the stomach unable to process several vitamins, leaves proteins only partially digested and a large number of minerals insoluble, so that they are lost and exit in waste matter. The consequences of this problem are also ballooning stomach gas and consequent pain.

So, in order for many other brain foods to be digested and absorbed, it is mandatory to take in sufficient vitamin B–1.

Niacin and Dilated Brain Capillaries

Like thiamine, vitamin B–3 (niacin) has a powerful influence on thinking and remembering. Niacin dilates arteries and capillaries in the brain, permitting greater entry of oxygen-carrying blood. So does the milder niacinamide, but to a lesser degree.

Professor Rudl Altschul, when chairman of the Department of Anatomy at the University of Saskatchewan, reviewed many studies of niacin. He claims that this vitamin, taken for several years, can reverse some atherosclerotic plaque in blood vessels. And I support him here.

A word of warning about niacin though. It can cause a flush, warmth, and itching or prickly skin for approximately 15 to 20 minutes. It's also best to take it with a B–complex supplement containing 50 to 100 milligrams of major B family members. My experience with patients is that niacinamide takes a little longer—often months longer—to restore memory.

Sustained release niacin has caused some liver damage; therefore, I do not advise using it. Large potencies of niacin should not be taken unless closely monitored by a knowledgeable health professional.

Over and above opening arteries wider, niacin helps to rejuvenate remembering and thinking for a very good reason. It is an important part of a coenzyme called NAD that helps to energize the brain. Insufficient niacin makes NAD incomplete so that it puts the biochemical brakes on metabolic reactions and interrupts the energy supply for brain cells.

The Trouble with Vitamin B–12

Best known of the B vitamin family for enhancing memory is vitamin B–12 (cyanocobalamin), the most complicated of all vitamins structurally. An experiment by Dr. A.J. MacDonald Holmes, reported in the *British Medical Journal,* demonstrated that a deficiency of cyanocobalamin can invite an array of mental and emotional problems: memory loss, difficulty in thinking, confusion, delusions, depression, and hallucinations.[4]

John Lindenbaum, M.D., of New York's Columbia-Presbyterian Medical Center and Harlem Hospital Center, validates the Holmes study.[5] Memory loss, tingling fingers and toes, walking difficulties, dementia, fatigue, and various neurological problems can indeed result from a deficiency of vitamin B–12.

Contrary to common medical opinion, as Dr. Lindenbaum indicates, individuals can also exhibit symptoms of nervous disorders from vitamin B–12 deficiency without presenting signs of anemia or overlarge red blood cells.

Unfortunately, vitamin B–12 is difficult to absorb. I call it "the reluctant vitamin," because your stomach must secrete enough of what is known as the "intrinsic factor" to overcome this problem. If your thyroid function is low, you may have difficulty absorbing it. Another researcher, Isobel Jennings, cites an experiment that makes this point.[6] Rats without thyroid glands didn't absorb vitamin B–12 at all.

Enough of my patients have had difficulty in absorbing vitamin B–12—even some supplemented with natural thyroid hormone—for me to recommend that they take one of two unconventional forms of this nutrient.

The first includes the intrinsic factor, and the other is sublingual B–12, tiny red pills that dissolve under your tongue. The latter enable the vitamin to take a direct route into the bloodstream.

Best dietary sources of cyanocobalamin, however, are fish, shellfish, liver and other organ meats, cheese, eggs, and legumes. Please be aware that cold water ocean fish avoid most manmade pollution. And don't forget that shellfish tend to congregate near the shore of bays, gulfs and oceans, where toxic pollutants collect.

It would seem logical that vitamin B–12 from foods would be best absorbed. This is what biochemists at the University of Southern California thought until a few years ago when they made a comparative test with human beings. Actually, vitamin B–12 supplements were better absorbed and assimilated.[7]

Choline: Memory Enhancer

Earlier we mentioned choline as a memory enhancer. In the early 1970s, for instance, biochemists theorized that choline is involved in learning and memory problems and that, as we age, we lose our ability to produce choline—itself a major reason for memory loss.[8]

These researchers also state that a study of young people whose choline-releasing ability was blocked suffered a memory loss, suggesting that the young people were aging prematurely.

An animal study by Dr. R.T. Bartus and associates also pointed to the effectiveness of choline for improving faulty memory.[9] Two groups of mice were tested for memory. One group was fed a choline-deficient diet. The other was put on a choline-enriched diet.

There was a decided difference between the two groups. Mice on the choline-enriched diet performed decidedly better than the choline-deprived mice. Old mice on the choline-enriched regimen performed as well as young mice. And choline-deprived young mice performed like old mice. Dr. Bartus repeated the experiment and came up with the same results and conclusion: Learning and memory are decidedly superior in choline-enriched mice than in choline-deficient mice. The same seems to hold true for humans.

Choline, of course, is a key ingredient in lecithin, a phospholipid found in soybeans, egg yolks, and liver with smaller amounts in fish and cereals. Lecithin is an emulsifier that breaks down fat. It is especially helpful in coping with fatty deposits in blood vessels.

In the brain it works this way. At the ends of certain brain cells choline changes into the neurotransmitter acetylcholine. Now choline in the blood comes from the diet—as lecithin or phosphatidylcholine—or from the liver where it is synthesized. Small amounts are secreted in brain cells. The liver's contribution of choline isn't quite enough for most bodies, so it is usually necessary to take a supplement—particularly as we age. Phosphatidylcholine is the best bet, because it has the highest concentration of choline.

Flexible Cell Membranes for Better Brains

In an Ohio State University study, mice fed lecithin or phosphatidylcholine showed a far better memory for solving the passages of a maze than unsupplemented mice. The bonus value was that their brains, viewed with high-powered instrumentation, seemed much younger. The cell membranes were far more flexible than those of the unsupplemented mice and with fewer fatty deposits.[10]

The aging brain becomes more rigid and clogged with fats, less able to take in nutrients efficiently and discharge wastes. This condition can cause memory loss and confused thinking.

Although we will write more about the merits of choline in the upcoming chapter on Alzheimer's disease, we must mention still another high-powered nutrient that revs up the memory and kicks thinking into high gear. We're talking about dimethylaminoethanol (DMAE). Here are just a few results of the many studies now being done on DMAE.

According to researcher R. Hochschild, DMAE readily reaches brain cell membranes and helps to renew them.[11]

Ross Pelton, Ph.D., remarks that DMAE rejuvenates the memory and boosts ability to learn and think efficiently.[12]

Dr. H.B. Murphree seconds the motion and adds that, over and above memory enhancement and more clear mental concentration, DMAE improves muscle tone and promotes better sleep.[13]

Other studies show that the neurotransmitter acetylcholine is nearly always deficient in memory loss and learning problems. DMAE enhances the production of choline, which is translated into acetylcholine that boosts memory and also uplifts mood and offers greater brain energy.[14] This is why supplementary DMAE is necessary.

Add to this the fact that it's difficult to take in enough DMAE in foods, because the few rich suppliers are sardines and anchovies, and we return to the need for supplements. How many of us eat sardines and anchovies daily?

Acetyl-L-Carnitine: Brain Booster Deluxe

Another nutrient doing spectacular things for deteriorating memory in the aged—even the young, for that matter—is acetyl-L-carnitine. This nutrient is to carnitine what Superman is to the average man. It does everything L-carnitine does, but better—such as moving fats across cell membranes into the mitochondria, energy producing mini-furnaces that super-charge brain and body cells.

Acetyl-L-carnitine's brain boosting was discovered by accident. Given to elderly patients for heart conditions, it improved mood, revived energy, and increased ability to think more clearly.

An Italian study also revealed an astonishing reversal of mental deterioration in the aged with acetyl-L-carnitine. As these researchers noted, the change was most notable in improved memory and "constructional thinking."[15]

Another Italian study, by biochemist A. Lino and associates, demonstrated that this nutrient accelerated reflex speed of teenagers and heightened their visual memory. As an added benefit, it extended the attention span of Down syndrome patients.[16]

Don't Overlook the Obvious

Pyroglutamic acid promotes brain energy and thinking and remembering. It was dramatically successful in coping with age-related memory decline—particularly verbal memory. This was proved with human as well as animal subjects.[17]

Well-known trace minerals such as boron and zinc also improve remembering and thinking.

One consideration often overlooked in memory flaws is concentration. For instance, we can't remember what we fail to take into our consciousness in the first place. Then as we age, many of us seem to observe less and then expect to remember.

In *Who Gets Sick* Dr. Blair Justice describes it this way:

> The remarkable ability of the brain to undergo physical changes in response to our perceived environments is providing new insights also into memory and learning.
>
> The synapses that connect each of our 100 billion neurons with as many as 50,000 brain cells can be deactivated or enhanced based on our experiences.[18]

In this light, if we observe ourselves trapped in a never-ending, gray environment (as in aging without remaining stimulated mentally and physically), our synapses can very well shut down and reduce the number of neurotransmitters.

This reaction is surely true about boron and the brain. James G. Penland, Ph.D., of the USDA's Human Research Center in Grand Forks, North Dakota, observes that a deficiency of boron changes brain waves—a drop in alpha wave activity—indicating a decline in alertness.[19]

"When you reduce dietary boron, you're almost certainly going to get a drop in alpha wave activity and an increase in theta wave activity from what we've seen on electroencephalograms (EEG)," writes Penland. "That's the same type of change you see when people become drowsy or less alert."

The Penland team fed women volunteers meals containing only 0.25 milligram of boron daily. At the halfway point of each study, a three milligram tablet of boron was added to make sure the women had an adequate intake of this trace mineral.

Boron is present in fruits and vegetables, so, for the sake of the study, meals omitted fruit and fruit juices and included only small portions of vegetables.

"Fast foods contain very little boron, even if they are accompanied by a lettuce and tomato salad," says Loanne Mullen, the dietician on the Penland team.

Tests showed reaction time of boron-deprived women to be slowed. "A lack of boron affects motor performance," states Dr. Penland.

Zinc's for the Memory. So Is Iron.

Like boron, both zinc and iron supplements cause impressive improvements in memory. Dr. Harold Sandstead's study done at the University of Texas Medical Branch at Galveston, revealed the towering importance of increasing the intake of these minerals.[20]

Inasmuch as one can easily upset the ratios of trace minerals to one another, it is best to take them under the guidance of a knowledgeable health professional.

Significant is the fact that 34 women between the ages of 18 and 40, with mild deficiencies of zinc and iron performed within normal range relative to memory, compared with 11 normal controls. However, when supplemented with either 30 milligrams of zinc or iron daily, they made gains up to 20 percent higher on standard memory tests, performing better than the controls.

Women who took both zinc and iron daily showed only a slight improvement in memory. Those on a multivitamin failed to improve. Why the minimal gain on both minerals? Dr. Sandstead explains that zinc and iron interfere with each other's absorption in supplements. However, they don't when a part of the entire diet.

He suggests that deficiencies of these minerals—and, therefore, a memory below potential—are caused because women avoid red meat, one of the best sources of both zinc and iron. Other good sources of these minerals are chicken, fish, beans, egg yolk, oats, blackstrap molasses, sunflower seeds, and wheat germ.

Dr. Sandstead suggests still another alternative, separating the minerals, taking one with breakfast and the other with dinner.

Memory Beyond Nutrients

Dozens of studies and many of my cases underscore the importance of healthful, natural foods and the proper supplements in enhancing memory. Still, it is also necessary to use memory properly. In helping my patients cope with what they call a "bad memory," I offer a formula that usually works.

First, I make sure that they are actually paying attention and taking in the information they want to remember. For instance, several patients complained about not remembering where their car was parked in a large shopping complex. Poor memory or poor observation? Most probably, they failed to note a parking lane number or other landmark in the line of sight of the aisle.

Incomplete observation usually leads to incomplete memory, frustration, and, in time, loss of confidence in your memory even if it is not to blame.

Make Memory a Game

What you do with information will also affect how well you remember it. One of my patients who couldn't remember jokes began to master them when I suggested he share them with family and friends. He suddenly had a deeper motivation.

It also helps to link new information to something you already know. Mnemonic devices are very helpful here. Named after Mnemosyne, the Greek goddess of memory, they were used thousands of years ago. The Greeks were quite fond of these memory prompts, and worked up formulas or systems for their use.

For example, it's easy to remember the name of a person named Green. You just visualize the color green. But how would you handle a more complicated name like Ashkenazy? You break it down into visual and audible segments, "ashcan-AH-Z."

How about Cunningham? Raymond Tucker, a Bowling Green State University professor who studies memory, would do it as follows: "sly pig." Now Mr. Cunningham might not enjoy the association, but it would get the job done for the person trying to recall his name.

How do you handle more numerous and less exotic names such as Jones, Smith, and Miller?

For Jones, you visualize a steaming cup of Joe (one of the slang terms for coffee) and add NZ. Smith is a cakewalk. You visualize The Village Smithy, little known today, except by the people who still own plow horses, racehorses, show horses, or polo horses and need a blacksmith to shoe their animals. Miller is a breeze, too. You see on your mind's screen an old mill on a stream turning grain into flour.

Memory wizard Hermione Hilton uses rhymes, some of them, silly, she admits. But who worries about "silly," if the devices work? "Mr. Hicks plays tricks." "Mr. Krause lives in a house." Or Mr. Krause could be a louse. Take your choice!

The name could be an occupation: Carpenter, Taylor, Barber, or Barker. It could be an object: Penney, as in (J.C.), Hamm, Slate, Kite, Coffey, or Calendar. Lots of people have brand names, as Ms. Hilton points out, such as Pillsbury, Campbell, Ford, Chrysler (spelled in different ways), Dodge, and, among others, Hoover.

Do you have trouble remembering whether the letter "i" comes before the letter "e"? Just recall the schoolkid's rhyme "i before e, except after c."

Remember how to recall the order of colors in the rainbow. Most schoolkids know the name Roy G. Biv—red, orange, yellow, green, blue, indigo, and violet.

And don't forget how to remember the number of days in each month: "Thirty days hath September, April, June and November. All the rest have 31, except February, which drew the short straw." Here's the best way to know how to set your clock for daylight saving time and then return it to standard time. "Spring ahead, Fall back."

Do you remember how to recall musical notes in the treble clef? "Every good boy does fine," or "Every good boy deserves fudge."

Now in schools, the teachers help students remember the position of the planets, according to their nearness to the sun: My Very Educated Mother Just Served Us Nine Pickles—Mercury, Venus, Earth, Mars, Jupiter, Saturn, Uranus, Neptune, and Pluto. Because two of the planets' names start with the letter M, they recall that Mercury comes first because it has more letters than Mars.

M.B. Grenier, teacher and memory buff, mentions a way to remember names of the Great Lakes—the word "homes": Huron, Ontario, Michigan, Erie, Superior.

You're ready to shop at the supermarket and don't want to make a list. Then use the Higbee system—that of Dr. Kenneth Higbee, a memory expert who taught psychology at Brigham Young University in Provo, Utah. You want to buy sweet rolls, milk, cereal, and pork chops. So you picture buns, sailing like a raft on a sea of milk, and a pair of shoes crunching through a field of cornflakes, and a tree with pork chops hanging from the branches like apples.

One of my elderly male patients resolved to improve his memory by memorizing with a purpose: sharing with friends useful tidbits of information that he gleaned from newspapers, magazines, and books. Soon they began complimenting him. This response fired him up with even more incentive.

He may not be the life of the party, but he has improved his memory vastly.

It is sad that so many people give up on their memory too early, especially with the thought that they are a victim of senile dementia or Alzheimer's disease. Worrying about it compounds the problem.

Most of the people who come to my office in desperation about what they call their lost memory usually find it again through natural foods, supplements mentioned in this book, thyroid supplementation, simple lifestyle changes, and physical and mental exercises. Soon their confidence is restored—their memory, too—and they can again enjoy living to the full!

CHAPTER 10

The Answers to Alzheimer's Disease?

With Alzheimer's disease, it's memory that almost always deteriorates first. Then judgment becomes impaired, followed by marked personality and temperament changes: irritability, hair-trigger temper, depression, nervousness, and anxiety.

Difficulty in thinking and speaking and inability to take care of personal needs are followed by humiliation that annihilates human dignity: inability to control the bladder and bowel and having to be diapered like a baby.

Among the four million Alzheimer's disease patients in the United States, some develop osteoporosis, or severe arthritis. Over a span of four to eight years, all of these symptoms worsen until once-feared death can seem merciful.

What causes Alzheimer's disease? There are almost as many theories about this as there are authorities on the subject. Some researchers point to the stress of environmental pollutants—mainly aluminum, the third most plentiful mineral in the earth's surface. Inasmuch as Alzheimer's disease victimizes mainly middle-agers to oldsters, other authorities believe that it is the aging process that makes people vulnerable. Others feel that marginal to extreme nutritional deficiency leaves some people open to the disease. Still others think it could be caused by free radical attack on the brain without enough opposing antioxidants, or it could even be caused by a weak immune system.

Of course, it could be every reason just mentioned—and some still unknown. But let's return for a moment to the environmental pollution theory, and the focus on aluminum. Is aluminum a cause—or *the* cause—or a by-product of the disease process?

In brain autopsies of numerous Alzheimer's disease victims, what do we find? A tangle of neurofibrils (nerve fibers, minute brain conductors), dead cells, and *aluminum* in the brain and spinal cerebrospinal fluid, plus deposits of amyloid—a waxy substance that comes from degenerated body tissues.

Evidence for the Aluminum Theory

Pinpointing aluminum as the major environmental cause for Alzheimer's is not a new idea. Almost 30 years ago, Dr. D. Crapper and associates at the University of Toronto, performed autopsies on numerous Alzheimer's patients.[1]

In every instance, they found aluminum in localized brain areas, amazing tangles of neurofibrils, as well as amyloid deposits. Several experiments revealed that when tiny amounts of aluminum were injected into the brains of laboratory animals, they invariably developed the tangled neurofibrils and the aluminum localized near them.

Donald R. McLaughlan, M.D., professor of physiology and medicine, and associates at the University of Toronto were some of those experimenters. They injected an infinitesimal amount of aluminum chloride (1 one-billionth of a mole) into the hippocampus area of a cat's brain.[2] The animal not only came down with Alzheimer's disease symptoms, but went through the entire sequence of symptoms, and then died.

The Answers to Alzheimer's Disease? 137

In a human study done at the Brain Bio Center in Princeton, New Jersey, 400 psychiatric patients with faulty memory and senile episodes were tested for blood levels of aluminum. Guess what? They were found to have much higher levels than nonpsychiatric patients.[3]

Aluminum also became a prime suspect some years ago in clinics for dialysis treatments. Municipal water used in this process brought on symptoms of senile dementia: failing memory, inability to think, dizziness, confusion, and other characteristics of a faltering, aged person.

Attendants discovered that when water used in dialysis had an elevated content of aluminum, symptoms of senile dementia increased. When it was low, symptoms of dementia declined.[4]

Can Aluminum Be Innocent?

Not long ago, the British government conducted a 10-year study of aluminum in drinking water in relation to 4,000 volunteers, ages 40 to 69, in 88 counties of England and Wales. Researchers compared the incidence of Alzheimer's disease with the levels of aluminum in the water supply of these areas.[5]

Their findings were not totally unexpected. Volunteers who drank water containing the most aluminum were calculated to have a 50 percent greater risk of developing Alzheimer's disease than those whose water was without aluminum.

One surprising discovery was that individuals under the age of 65 are at much greater risk—in fact, 70 percent more likely—of developing Alzheimer's disease than older persons, if their drinking water contains a high level of aluminum. What was the researchers' definition of a "high" level? It was 0.11 milligrams per liter of water.

How does aluminum get into water supplies aside from that leached from the earth as water collects in reservoirs? Most municipal water plants use a form of aluminum, alum, a white, powdery, evaporating substance to settle sediment. You'll also find alum listed on the label of almost all bottled dill pickles in supermarkets.

Most processed foods contain some form of aluminum, too: free-flowing salt, some white flour or bread and pastries made from it, most baking powders, many salad dressings, fruit and vegetable juices, and soft drinks in aluminum cans.

Although natural cheese may contain one-half to three milligrams of aluminum per gram, processed cheese may contain as much as 144 milligrams per gram.

Many commonly used products contain aluminum that stealthily invades your mind and body. (Please read labels carefully.) You'll find it listed in many acne medications, antacids, antidiarrhea products, antiperspirants, buffered aspirin, deodorants, some cosmetics, douches and other feminine products, certain hemorrhoid preparations, lipstick, skin creams, lotions, and even certain toothpastes. Aluminum is also in cigarette filters, food wrappers, and the foil in which some people save and refrigerate leftover foods.

Fluoride and Aluminum: A Double Threat

For years, many studies have revealed the health hazards of cooking with aluminum pots and pans. The hazard is especially acute if your community supplies fluoridated water. In this regard, we turn to Dr. Richard P. Murray, who cites a study conducted by the Department of Biochemistry at Sri Lanka University.[6]

When fluoridated water was boiled in an aluminum pan, the pan released 0.2 part per million (ppm) within 10 minutes. The higher the fluoride content of water, the more aluminum was released.

When water with a one percent addition of fluoride is boiled in an aluminum pan for 10 minutes, it releases the frightening amount of 200 ppm. Even more frightening is the fact that, in 1986, the Environmental Protection Agency authorized an increase in the addition of fluoride to public water supplies from one part per million to as much as four parts.

Fluoride doesn't need aluminum to be toxic. As little as one part per million has been shown in several studies to impair the biological efficiency of the brain's acetylcholine by as much as 61 percent. Remember that acetylcholine is the main neurotransmitter involved in memory, attention span, and thinking.

Further, fluoride threatens us in more than the water supply: in sodas, beer, fruit and vegetable juices processed in communities that fluoridate water, in canned, boxed, bottled processed foods, and in toothpastes and mouthwashes. Pressure on the Food and Drug Administration finally led to this government body's requirement that toothpaste companies put a warning about fluoride on its products' containers.

Fortunately, every toiletry and food product mentioned above can be bought at health food stores minus the aluminum and fluoride. Also, spring water without fluoride is available in supermarkets as well as in health food stores.

Many individuals treat the fluoride issue lightly. They don't realize that fluoride was once the most effective rat poison on the market. Fluoride is a by-product in the making of synthetic fertilizers and the processing of aluminum. This waste product had no place to go until someone came up with the bright idea of saving the teeth of the world's children by fluoridating water. But even if the teeth of children in communities with fluoridated water are more cavity-free than those of kids in nonfluoridated areas—and there are studies to dispute this—is it worth the greater risk?

A Polluted Person

One of my elderly women patients who lived in a water-fluoridated community where alum was also used was brought to my offices by her daughter. She was stupefied, dizzy, unable to keep her balance without help, weak, and unable to remember much of anything.

I knew immediately that she needed detoxification and no fewer than eight glasses daily of *only* bottled spring water, an upgraded diet and nutritional supplements. That is what I recommended for her.

After in-depth questioning, I learned that she took aluminum-laden antacids with orange juice. A study I had just come across revealed that the acidity of citrus juices increases absorption of aluminum by ten times. I asked her to stop this practice.

Suspecting that her intestinal distress was caused not by too much stomach acid, but by too little, I had her take a test to learn her status. It turned out she wasn't secreting enough hydrochloric acid and digestive enzymes.

I also had her follow a special regimen shared with me by the late Dr. Carl Pfeiffer, of the Brain Bio Center: a phosphate-rich diet that helps draw aluminum out of the system. Best food bets for phosphates are almonds, bran flakes, brewer's yeast, kidney beans, lentils, liver, peanuts, pumpkin seeds, sesame seeds, and soybeans. (Please don't forget the warning about peanuts and the carcinogenic aflatoxin mold on some crops.)

Her daughter promised to make sure her mother followed my regimen. She did. Within six months, the change in her was remarkable. She had worked wonders by drinking abundant pure spring water daily, eating only natural foods and taking a daily multipurpose vitamin-mineral supplement, along with hydrochloric acid and digestive enzymes.

Six months later, my elderly patient walked briskly into my office without her daughter's help. She looked 10 years younger. Her energy and memory had returned as her dizziness had vanished. She was again optimistic and determined. She even wanted to go back to work.

Another Way for Aluminum to Invade Us

Although you can sometimes reduce elevated blood levels of aluminum by taking zinc, magnesium, and manganese supplements, this still may not address its removal from brain cells. It's worth a try, but prevention is the best route to follow in any case.

No matter what regimen you may follow, it's virtually impossible to escape all aluminum. There are even aluminum particulates in the very air we breathe. Want to know more? Let's hear from Dr. Stephen Davies, director of the Biolab Medical Unit in London and a world authority on personal toxicity.

Over seven years, Dr. Davies measured the amount of aluminum, lead, cadmium, arsenic and mercury in the blood of 3,000 patients, in the sweat of 15,000 patients, and in the hair of 17,000 patients. As Dr. Davies reaffirmed:

> ... such progressive increases in human heavy-metal toxicity come from the inhalation of fine metallic particulates and other air pollutants. He condemned aluminum air particulates as the most noteworthy potential source of dementia pathology.[7]

There's no mystery about how aluminum gets into our body. We cannot completely avoid it as long as we insist on eating, drinking, and breathing. For many years, medical opinion held that little, if any, aluminum could enter the bloodstream through the digestive tract. This is why many doctors felt it was safe to prescribe antacids and other medicines containing aluminum.

An Eye-Opening Study

Certainly aluminum couldn't find a way through the protective blood–brain barrier! So how does aluminum do the impossible? Quite easily. Aluminum ions are tiny. They are not quite half the size of ions of minerals essential to the body and mind: calcium, magnesium, potassium, and sodium.[8]

Experiments by researchers at the University of Virginia at Charlottesville have led them to a theory that explains how aluminum damages the brain. Timothy L. MacDonald, W. Griffith Humphreys, and R. Bruce Martin have discovered that aluminum undermines structures called microtubules that support brain and body cells.[9]

Filaments called spindles are formed from these microtubules. Cells can't divide without them. Nothing is status quo with microtubules. They are ever-active, being assembled and being taken apart. They are made with a raw material called tubulin, amino acids, and magnesium.

Here's how aluminum undermines the structure of tubulin. Receptors on the tubulin are supposed to accept magnesium exclusively. As they don't discriminate, aluminum competes for vacant sites.

Aluminum has an advantage over magnesium. It enters tubulin 10 times faster than magnesium, thus occuping more sites. Since aluminum is not as strong a component as magnesium, the tubulin structure can weaken to the point of collapse.

Does Alzheimer's Disease Disconnect Memory?

If this research is correct, it still doesn't explain how tangled neurofibrils destroy memory. Researcher Bradley T. Hyman and his team at the University of Iowa at Iowa City conducted an in-depth investigation to solve this mystery. They discovered that tangled nerve fibers near the deposits of aluminum are distributed within layers of cells that serve as relays for nerve impulses into and out of the brain's memory center.[10]

The Answers to Alzheimer's Disease?

General opinion holds that the biochemical damage done by Alzheimer's disease is mainly *in* the hippocampus, where many memories are recorded. The Hyman team found that the nerve-tangle damage was in the area *surrounding* the hippocampus.

Hyman observes that these blockages cut off input and output from the hippocampus. It is not that memory is lost, he says. It is as if the phone lines are cut off.

These two studies give clear signals that aluminum is not the kind of mineral that anyone would want to host in mind or body. But is there a reliable way to get rid of it?

A Compelling Case for Chelation

"Yes," maintains Richard Casdorph, M.D., of Long Beach, California, who has had phenomenal success with chelation treatments in patients in early or mid-stage Alzheimer's disease.[11]

The case of Robert, a once bright and creative 57-year-old chemical engineer, is particularly fascinating. After 30 years with a major chemical company, he was forced to take disability retirement because his memory had deteriorated.

Several medical centers, including that of Johns Hopkins University School of Medicine, had diagnosed him as an Alzheimer's disease patient. His wife, Cynthia, took him to a local neurologist to confirm the diagnosis, which a blood–brain flow study corroborated. The neurologist then told Cynthia that no treatment would help.

Agatha, Robert's mother, thought differently. She had heard of Dr. Casdorph's success with chelation and offered to pay for her son's treatment.

After Robert had a thorough physical, Dr. Casdorph requested that he submit to a psychometric exam—including a memory and I.Q. test—by an independently practicing local psychologist. Results showed a significant reduction in brain function from Robert's normal level. As a baseline study, it verified unequivocally his diagnosis of Alzheimer's disease.

Dr. Casdorph started Robert on chelation but without quick improvement. Then, after three months, a normal period in chelation therapy, Robert's memory began to return. Soon thereafter, he was doing the kinds of everyday tasks that were so recently beyond him. Thirty sessions later, Agatha noted a marked improvement in Robert's thinking and remembering, and in his physical health. Soon his mind and memory were nearly back to normal. He even began bicycling and cross-country hiking again.

Chelation treatments had removed his heavy metal accumulation caused by having worked at a chemical company for 30 years. Finally, after 63 chelations, Robert again went through psychometric testing. The psychologist reported that his I.Q. had risen by 13 percent, and his memory score by 12 percent.

Soon the patient who had been diagnosed as incurable was pronounced cured. Agatha, Robert's mother, was so impressed that she elected to have a physical evaluation and chelation treatments by Dr. Casdorph herself.

I do know this: If I or my loved ones were diagnosed with Alzheimer's disease, I would surely elect for chelation. Despite the bad rap that some doctors give to chelation, there is no downside for it—only an upside. If the candidate fails the mandatory, pre-chelation test of the kidneys—meaning their function can't throw off wastes etched into the arteries—he or she is not permitted to take chelation.

Another Approach to Alzheimer's Disease

Are there any other ways of coping with Alzheimer's disease? The nutritional supplement choline, one of the B vitamins, has proved helpful. The brain converts choline into acetylcholine, the chemical exuded between nerve cells to make thinking and remembering possible.

Some alternative doctors recommend that their senile dementia or Alzheimer's disease patients take supplements such as choline, acetylcholine, or lecithin that contains choline.[12]

For example, in a six months' study in London, Alzheimer's disease patients were given large doses of lecithin. Fifty percent of these patients improved in memory, thinking, and ability to care for their personal needs as a result.

Richard Wurtman, M.D., of MIT, an eminent authority on the biochemistry of the brain, in one study found a possible major reason for deterioration of memory: the amount of the neurotransmitter acetylcholine made from choline seems to be depleted by up to 90 percent from normal in Alzheimer's disease patients.[13]

Aside from a faulty memory, Alzheimer's disease patients often have behavioral problems, making them difficult to handle, a prime reason why many need professional care.

Test results of Dr. Raymond Levy, a University of London brain researcher, who gave choline therapy to 24 Alzheimer's disease patients, are noteworthy here. Eight patients showed definite and continued behavioral improvement—a remarkable result, even if it does not appear so numerically.[14]

Patients who improved averaged 79 years of age. Patients who failed to improve averaged 69 years of age. Dr. Levy's conclusion? Choline therapy is apparently most effective from a behavioral standpoint in individuals who develop Alzheimer's disease in the late-in-life years or in patients who have a mild form of this ailment.

Another Plausible Theory

Research by Neil R. Sims, M.D., at the Burke Rehabilitation Center in White Plains, New York, convinces him that Alzheimer's disease patients deteriorate not so much from lack of dietary raw materials such as lecithin or choline, as from another cause.[15] As they age, such patients lose their ability to synthesize acetylcholine from these raw materials.

This also appears to be the reason why lecithin is more effective in coping with Alzheimer's disease in its early stages, prior to the time that the ability to make acetylcholine slows or shuts down completely.

In this regard, Dr. Brian L.G. Morgan offers his approach to dealing with Alzheimer's disease: one to two grams of choline daily or 30 grams of lecithin. Best results occur when supplementing with lecithin that is 100 percent phosphatidylcholine.[16]

A revealing study by Dr. Judith Marquis in the Department of Pharmacology at Boston University throws more light on understanding Alzheimer's disease and how to moderate or even prevent it.[17]

Marquis discovered that aluminum seems to block the metabolism of acetylcholine. If it can't be metabolized, it is not available as a neurotransmitter to communicate information that makes thinking or remembering possible. Marquis also discovered this curious fact: Being well nourished with calcium limits the amount of aluminum that can accumulate in critical areas of the brain.

Other possible means of delaying or even blocking the onset of Alzheimer's disease may come through consuming lycopene-containing vegetables and fruit—tomatoes, watermelon, pink grapefruit, and guava. Lycopene, one of the powerful antioxidants that protects against most cancers and heart disease, is found most abundantly in the red coloring substance in tomatoes.

For his part, Robert C. Atkins, M.D., noted internationally for his beliefs in preventive medicine, calls lycopene "perhaps the strongest and most underrated carotenoid." What Atkins means, of course, is that lycopene is usually not as well known as its biochemical cousin beta-carotene.

Another study, this time of aged Catholic sisters in Mankato, Minnesota, also indicates that blood levels of lycopene are low in Alzheimer's disease patients. Some of the sisters in the study were in their mid-nineties with a few pushing the 100 year mark.[18]

Sisters with the highest blood levels of lycopene retained their memory longer and were able to take care of their personal needs for many more years than those with low levels of lycopene. Sisters with the lowest blood levels of lycopene were most Alzheimer's disease-prone. More about this remarkable nutrient in Chapter 13.

Excellent progress has been made in helping patients cope with Alzheimer's disease, particularly with chelation therapy and the use of the supplements lecithin, choline, and phosphatidylcholine. Fortunately, the outlook is improving even more.

CHAPTER 11

Hormones for the Head

In the beauty salon, talk about hormones is usually focused on sex, menstrual problems, menopause, and living longer. In the locker room, it's usually limited to sex, muscle building, and living longer.

Today it's no longer business as usual. In both places, talk about hormones is moving into an additional area: using them to stay physically *and* mentally young.

That's what this chapter is all about.

Four steroid hormones in particular will be featured: pregnenolone, dehydroepiandrosterone (DHEA), melatonin, and human growth hormone. The first three are available in health food stores. Human growth hormone can be obtained with a doctor's prescription. It is best to take hormones under the guidance of a physician well versed in their use.

Pregnenolone is first because it is the initial hormone that the body develops on the way to making steroid hormones. It comes mainly from cholesterol. It is called pregnenolone, because—in a certain sense—it is the mother who gives birth to dehydroepiandrosterone (DHEA) from its raw materials.

DHEA is an only child, but it, in turn, produces offspring,

passing along some of its raw materials that become the sex hormones, estrogen and testosterone, the biochemical grandchildren of pregnenolone.

According to William Regelson, M.D., a foremost authority on the subject from the Medical College of Virginia, Virginia Commonwealth University, both the adrenal cortex and the brain make pregnenolone.[1]

As with other hormones, we produce less and less of pregnenolone as we age. Eventually we are faced with a choice: take supplementary pregnenolone to remain mentally and physically young longer or do nothing and live with the consequences.

The Bright Promise of Pregnenolone

After hearing of pregnenolone's remarkable effects, one of my patients asked the logical question, "Where has it been all my life?"

The truth of the matter is pregnenolone has been with her and the rest of us all of our lives, and in human beings since the beginning of time. We've just been hearing more about it lately. Research that dates back to the middle 1940s showed that pregnenolone boosts the ability to learn and to remember.

During the same period, research indicated that pregnenolone might be helpful in coping with spinal cord injuries and in offering relief from rheumatoid arthritis: less pain, more mobility, and less fatigue. True enough, it was not an instant healer of this kind of arthritis, but it worked well over several months.

Ray Sahelian, M.D., in his book *Pregnenolone,* relates results of a study in this area. Back in 1950, a researcher named Henderson gave 21 patients 100 milligrams of pregnenolone acetate for five to 30 days. He followed up with 100 milligrams one to three times a week. Out of the entire group eight patients showed a dramatic improvement, four benefited moderately, four improved slightly, and four showed no change.[2]

So what happened to the hormone and its hopeful use as a supplement? Two things: As a natural substance secreted by the body, it was not patentable, so no drug company wanted to fund research or pursue the FDA's tedious approval process. Then about the same time, synthetic cortisone hit the market and cornered the rheumatoid arthritis therapy industry. Before the paeans of praise for cortisone died down, its horrendous side effects had already turned off medical doctors and patients. This "miracle cure" brought on a greater incidence of osteoporosis and diabetes, water retention, high blood pressure, and puffiness of the tissues, causing "moon face."

Enhances Memory

Only in the last decade has interest in pregnenolone revived—this time for boosting memory and brain function.

How good a memory booster is pregnenolone? Phenomenal! Take it from two of the most prominent pregnenolone researchers, Eugene Roberts, Ph.D., of the City of Hope in Duarte, California, and John E. Morley, M.D., of the University of St. Louis.

One of Dr. Roberts' earliest animal pregnenolone studies, in 1992, demonstrated that this hormone is 100 times more powerful in improving the memory than any other substance.[3]

Dr. Morley, a coworker in this experiment, was equally extravagant in his praise:

> It is by far the most potent of the neurosteroids for improving memory by light years, and it has a much broader memory response than any of the other neurosteroids. This makes it almost an ideal agent for

looking at memory and the consequences of the age-related deterioration of memory.[4]

Like a sudden spectacular lightning flash, an animal experiment several years ago illuminated the minds of biochemists and psychologists to the potential of pregnenolone for boosting memory and thinking power.

Researcher J.F. Flood and associates, used only a picomolar amount of pregnenolone in rats—the approximate size of a pinpoint.[5]

Placed in a T-shaped maze, the rats were supposed to find the correct arm of the maze for their "reward." If they didn't end up in the right arm within five seconds, they experienced a slight electric shock after each try until they succeeded.

After performing the test successfully, they were tested again within a week to determine how well they had learned the maze and how to avoid their shocking experience. A majority of rats were given one of several steroids or a placebo (a look-alike "nothing" treatment).

Each of the hormones lowered the number of runs needed to relearn the most efficient route to destination, improving their shock-avoidance performance. But pregnenolone gave rats the best results at 1 one-hundredth (1/100) the potency of hormones administered to others!

Almost Unbelievable

Another unusual factor about pregnenolone is that it possibly can enhance your memory *after the fact*.[6] Say that you learned the names of 12 people at a party today. Then tomorrow you were given a capsule of pregnenolone. That capsule supposedly would make you better able to remember those names than if you hadn't taken it.

Several animal studies validated this finding, at least potentially for humans. Dr. Eugene Roberts, a noted researcher in the field, believes, however, that the studies will prove to be true for you and me, as well.[7] Roberts is a man of his word and has initiated studies with human beings.

If you find anecdotal reports of importance—and I do—then the evidence is mounting. I also speak from personal experience here. Several of my senior citizen patients who have tried pregnenolone (in one 50 milligram capsule daily, best taken before breakfast), tell me they noted a definite memory improvement. There is something else here, too. They believed that by taking the hormone, they achieved a greater feeling of tranquillity—of peace of mind.

One patient reported improved powers of observation and the ability to see many more details in a natural setting—anywhere, for that matter—that he had never before noted. It was almost as if his awareness had taken a photograph, capturing the most minute details. This image reminded me of an FBI man I met years ago who told me that part of his training had been to stand in front of a variety store's display window for only a few seconds and then be able to name every item shown.

A New Level of Consciousness

This patient's experience is somewhat similar to that reported by Dr. Sahelian, when he increased his personal dosage of pregnenolone to 30 milligrams daily.[8] While strolling on the beachfront walk in Venice, California, he felt a mild euphoria, as he reports:

> I became more conscious of my surroundings. Flowers growing in the front gardens of the ocean homes seemed brighter and prettier.... A mosaic on the door of a beach house caught my eye. Examining it closer, I noticed that it was a scene of tall redwood trees with a curving blue stream running through the middle....

It dawned on me that I had walked by this house many times without paying attention to this artwork. Everything seemed to be more beautiful and intriguing....

Inasmuch as I am blessed with a fairly good memory, I had not tried pregnenolone until I read the above words by Dr. Sahelian. Now I know it works!

So far as memory is concerned, dehydroepiandrosterone (DHEA), the hormone that follows pregnenolone in the biological sequence, also seems to produce similar reactions to those evoked by pregnenolone.

In several mouse studies, for instance, DHEA definitely enhanced memory which encouraged Dr. Eugene Roberts and others to continue experiments in the hope that it will benefit human beings as well.

A New Memory for an Old One

Can you exchange a new memory for an old one? Some researchers seem to think so. But how, in fact, can this happen?

High levels of DHEA are in the brain. Low levels are associated with fewer brain neurons and fewer neurotransmitters such as acetylcholine, norepinephrine, and serotonin and, consequently, reduced ability of brain cells to communicate with one another. The result: undependable memory, difficulty in concentrating, depression, poor muscle coordination, and difficulty in falling asleep and staying asleep.

DHEA supplementation, along with vitamin B–complex, additional choline, and pantothenic acid—as well as the amino acids, phenylalanine, tryptophan, and tyrosine—can enhance and increase the making of neurotransmitters. Only in one particular area do the benefits from pregnenolone and DHEA overlap: enhancing memory. And pregnenolone shows some superiority there and in coping with rheumatoid arthritis. Some alternative and complementary doctors are also treating asthma, lupus, and multiple sclerosis with pregnenolone.

For my patients taking 25 milligrams of DHEA daily, clearer thinking and improved memory, better sleeping, and a feeling of greater energy are common. My colleagues in preventive medicine also have much good to say about their DHEA results with patients:

"Seems to upgrade the memory!"

"Reduced the weight of a patient who stayed on her same caloric intake."

"Increased the energy of several patients."

"Improved the sex life of an intermittently impotent patient."

"Restored memory and the patient's confidence in his ability to give talks to the public."

Human Growth Hormone: Incredible Results

Another key hormone that appears to improve thinking and remembering is human growth hormone (hGH). It has also shown spectacular results in renewing vitality of middle-agers and the elderly, improving strength, contributing to weight reduction and muscle-building, strengthening the immune system, lowering blood pressure, and enhancing—sometimes reviving—sexual performance.

Dr. Ronald Klatz, president of the American Academy of Anti-Aging Medicine, told an audience of physicians that hGH has worked revival wonders in many individuals. It has reversed brain shrinkage, typical of mid-lifers and the elderly, has accelerated reaction time and ability to take in new information, mental alertness, and renewed ability to remember.[9]

In his talk, Dr. Klatz discussed rat experiments in which growth hormone improved myelin sheaths protecting cells, making them even better insulators of nerves. When myelin breaks down, it brings on devastating illnesses such as multiple sclerosis.

In laboratory cells, hGH did the impossible: synthesizing RNA, the messengers that carry out DNA instructions for the fissioning of new cells. Dr. Klatz states that this can happen in adult brains—that hGH can actually "stimulate cell division, repair and rejuvenation."[10]

Referring to the rat experiments of Dr. Marian Diamond, mentioned in Chapter 2, Dr. Klatz explained that when brains of her rats increased in size, it was not the brain cells themselves that increased. It was the dendrites, the tree-like extensions of the cells that grew. You will remember that Dr. Diamond helped dendrites expand by supplying rats with a stimulating environment—new toys daily and companions. So apparently similar results can be realized by giving rats growth hormone.

Equally remarkable is a discovery by Sam Baxas, of Baxamed Clinic in Switzerland, as related in Dr. Ronald Klatz's book, *Grow Young with hGH*.[11] Dr. Baxas, who has used human growth hormone for almost 25 years, placed brain and body cells in a petri dish and witnessed that they stopped dividing. Then he added growth hormone, and the cells started dividing again. He believes that further tests in vivo will show just how well hGH can slow down aging and even reverse aging to some extent.[12]

The Transformation of Dr. John Baron

Dr. Klatz also features a fascinating case study in his book—that of John Baron, a doctor of osteopathy and director of the Baron Clinic and American Institute of Anti-Aging in Cleveland.[13] Always in great shape physically, attributable to nutritional and vitamin programs for the last 50 years, Dr. Baron added growth hormone to his regimen less than two years ago. Klatz paints a colorful charaterization of Dr. Baron.

"At age eighty-two, John Baron looks about sixty and has the endurance of an Energizer bunny."

Dr. Baron who can still do exercises that would challenge a forty-year-old, comments on hGH:

"The most dramatic changes I noticed were in my energy, concentration and memory—both short and long term—and enhanced creativity."

Even that's not the end of the Baron story. Dr. Baron's waist narrowed from 44 inches to 38 when he was on growth hormone, although his weight remained the same: 189 pounds. His facial and body skin tightened. His face looks more youthful and his hair stopped graying. It even began growing back where he had bald spots. His failing distant vision improved so much that he longer needs glasses for driving.

One of the big surprises was the return of his sexual capabilty. "It's as good as it was when I was twenty-five," he claims.

The pituitary gland's output of growth hormone declines mainly because of lifestyle body-mind insults—alcohol, cigarettes, recreational drugs, overeating and various other stresses—rather than because of passing years.

The Klatz book also mentions research of Jan Berend Deijen and other Dutch scientists at the Free University Hospital in Amsterdam.[14] Studying male patients, Deijen discovered that those who were low in growth hormone reflected this deficiency in their declining mental ability and faulty memory.

Specifically, deficiency in growth hormone showed in the capability of processing a flash of information (called iconic memory), short-term memory, long-term memory, and what we call perceptual motor skills such as hand-eye coordination.

Other researchers worldwide are proving that, by supplementing deficient growth hormone to the appropriate levels, adults improve in their ability to think and reason.

Why the Opposition to Growth Hormone?

It is standard procedure for the orthodox mind to denigrate the new. And such a mind has a bit of ammunition to work with about the dangers of human growth hormone.

Those who oppose something as revolutionary as hGH injections for purposes of rejuvenation point to the early studies of hGH, during which there were many stunning successes and a few unpleasant side effects. Throughout the history of medicine, there have been negatives and failures in the early uses of drugs and hormones. This was true of thyroid hormone, of the first chelations, even of early administration of certain vitamin supplements.

Once the mistakes were corrected, these innovations proved to be safe and advanced the cause of preventive medicine and promoted improved health. The July 5, 1990, issue of the *New England Journal of Medicine,* the Rolls-Royce of medical publications, ran the story of the initial study with hGH done by Daniel Rudman, M.D., and colleagues at the Medical College of Wisconsin.[15]

An earthquake of the magnitude of 9 on the Richter scale rocked the medical research world when Rudman boldly stated:

"The effects of six months of human growth hormone on lean body mass and adipose tissue were equivalent in magnitude to the changes incurred during 10 to 20 years of aging."

The sin that Daniel Rudman had committed was being revolutionary, and, not content with being revolutionary, he had claimed the "impossible"—making his volunteers 10 to 20 years younger.

Here are the main points of the Rudman study of 12 diverse men from 61 to 81 years of age. Many were flabby with bulging bellies and love handles. They were injected with growth hormone for six months. hGH worked a near magic transformation, turning them into more slender, energetic, more mentally alert, and younger individuals.[16]

Reporters from every branch of the media flocked to the scene to witness these miracles. Gray hair of a now-bouncy 65-year-old had started turning black. A man too weak to unscrew the lid of a mayonnaise jar was now opening them with ease. Wrinkles on the hands of one member of the Golden Years gang had disappeared. A wife complained about not being able to keep up with her newly energized spouse. When the talk shifted to sexual competency, there were backhanded references about the return of youthfulness in the bedroom.

Naturally, for purposes of scientific legitimacy, Dr. Rudman had a control group in the study. And there they were with their flab and bulges in all the old familiar places and the same amount of ballast. There was no shift to lean body mass. They all looked and acted as old as they were, all aging in accordance with their lifestyle indiscretions and stresses.

Rudman's Remarkable Follow-Up Study

Despite the expected flak from orthodox researchers, Dr. Rudman did a follow-up study with 26 elderly volunteers. After complete physicals to establish baselines, the men were administered hGH, and the results were virtually the same.[17]

Rudman found that livers, spleens, and muscles that had withered returned to sizes typical of youthful men. Rudman pointed out that growth hormone could turn the bedridden into ambulatory patients or ex-patients, could enable the helpless to care for themselves again, and could help to slash the nation's mushrooming medical bill.

Soon other scientists worldwide were researching as Rudman had done, and some found side effects. Patients developed bones that were oversized for their sockets or bones in the head were misshaped. Other cases of carpal tunnel syndrome appeared as well.

Perhaps the future holds other similar mistakes in store for us. But researchers are learning from them, proceeding with more caution, tempering dosages, and approaching the problem slowly—to do less in more time and to be safe in the bargain.

Young Again in Palm Springs

Now for a success story based on Jim Scheer's interview with the world's most successful medical doctor in administering growth hormone treatments. This is Edmund Chein, M.D., head of the Palm Springs Life Extension Institute in the southern California desert community of Palm Springs, the wintertime mecca of sun worshipers galore.

Dr. Chein, a rehabilitation specialist, has never had a mishap with more than 1,000 patients. And he sees no need for one. He has had only successes in body and mind youthification.

Dr. Chein became a believer when he began fearing the consequences of his own out-of-condition physique, including an enlarged prostate. Overweight with a large pot belly, his cholesterol and triglyceride levels out of sight, and beginning to experience chest pains, he went to a doctor.

Familiar with the Rudman studies, Dr. Chein refused the conventional route—synthetic drugs to lower his cholesterol and triglycerides and a coronary bypass. Instead, he would try growth hormone on himself before he would try it on patients.

Down through the ages, doctors have used a similar method of experimentation. Hippocrates, the ancient Greek Father of Medicine, did so by using remedies on himself before giving them to patients. Much later, Samuel Hahnemann (1755–1843), a German physician, tried homeopathic remedies on himself and family before treating patients with them. Today homeopathic medicine is growing worldwide.

Dr. Chein was no different. First a physician friend tested Chein's hormone levels: thyroid, testosterone, DHEA, and growth hormone. All were low, and Dr. Chein decided to try hormone replacement to the level of a twenty-year-old. Within six months, his cholesterol and triglyceride levels had plummeted to normal. The big belly became a small flat belly, his flesh became more firm, and the chest pains disappeared along with the enlargement of his prostate.

The doctor who treated Dr. Chein was so impressed with the improvements that he also put himself on the growth hormone regimen—in fact, on the full range of hormone replacement—and soon he, too, experienced positive changes.

As a result, Dr. Chein opened the Palm Springs Life Extension Institute and prides himself on not having a failure in six years of rejuvenation experience. "It's a slam dunk, if you know what you're doing," he says.

All of his success is not based on hGH therapy alone. It is imperative, he states, to bring all hormone levels up, along with hGH.

Dr. Chein's Procedure

His secret? Starting with fundamentals. A thorough physical exam determines the state of health and the total hormone status of patients, not just for that of hGH. Using this as a baseline, he compensates for all hormonal deficiencies. Then he begins hGH treatments with low dosages of hGH.

Soon his patients administer the hormone to themselves

on six out of seven days at the times when the body customarily secretes it: just before bedtime at night and upon getting up in the morning. At first some patients shudder at the thought of injecting themselves. This was a fear of Bob Jones, who is in his late 60s and now looks as if he's in his early 40s. He told Jim Scheer:

> Your imagination runs wild. You visualize a needle the diameter of a telephone pole. And it's not like that at all. It's so small that you hardly feel it. I'm so glad I took the whole course of Dr. Chein's treatment.

Early in establishing his Institute, Dr. Chein worked in conjunction with L. Cass Terry, M.D., Ph.D., chairman and professor of neurology at the Medical College of Wisconsin in Milwaukee. Dr. Terry was an associate of the late Dr. Rudman.

Together the doctors wrote a comprehensive report on the first one thousand patients treated with hGH and other hormones. Dr. Chein has had an amazing success rate in every area of illness related to aging: improvements in strength, ability to exercise, and body fat, in skin and hair, in healing, flexibility, and resistance, sexual function, energy, emotions, and memory range from a low of 39 percent to a high of 88 percent. In most cases, the improvement in ability to think and remember has been astonishing.

Although most of Dr. Chein's initial studies were with men, he treats women just as readily and has a similar success rate with them.

The Doctor Offers an Incredible Guarantee

A common fear of new patients is the possibility of growth hormone causing cancer. This has not happened to any of Dr. Chein's patients. Further, he has seen several reversals of cancers, including prostate cancer and a reduction to normal of elevated prostate specific antigens (PSA) readings.

Dr. Chein's 100 percent success rate is going to continue, he says. From top TV, film, stage, and sports stars being treated by him with hGH and other hormones, he has an amazingly thick sheaf of testimonial letters. Promises he makes to patients are hard to believe, but here's what he said to Jim Scheer:

> I tell my patients if I can't get the blood level of your hormones to look like that of a 20-year-old, you can have your money refunded.
>
> I also have a guarantee for those with osteoporosis: a gain in bone density of 1.5 to 2.5 percent every six months, as shown by means of a bone scan. For those carrying around more weight than they want, I guarantee a weight loss of 10 to 12 percent of body fat every six months. Also, the changes in body fat to lean mass ratio will continue until the body composition has returned to that of a twenty-year-old.

Although Dr. Chein attracts patients from every continent in the world, there are some individuals who can't fly, drive, or bus to Palm Springs, California.

"No problem," says Dr. Chein. "I send or fax the person a list of lab tests that have to be done to establish a baseline. Any legitimate lab in the world can perform these tests."

Test results can be faxed or mailed to Dr. Chein's offices. Then he determines the mix of hormones needed and sends it to patients, along with a videotape of his procedures.

Dr. Chein also lends a video camera to distant patients. With camera plugged into a computer, he and patients can talk face to face, seeing and hearing one another. He can also demonstrate how and where on the body patients are to inject the human growth hormone. Now, thanks to the computer age, patients in any part of the world can be treated by Dr. Chein.

Preventive medicine and alternative doctors capable of following his protocol are now all over the world. When Jim Scheer talked with Dr. Chein, he had just returned from Hong Kong, where he gave an in-depth seminar to train doctors there in his methods.

When patients first hear of Dr. Chein's results with the hormone treatment, they are reluctant to believe them. However, those who visit Dr. Chein's offices and view "before" and "after" photos of patients—or meet them in person—are amazed and usually have a one word comment: "Wow!"

CHAPTER 12

How to Raise Your Child's I.Q.—Part One

The best time to prepare to boost your child's I.Q. is about two years before he or she is born! The next best time is nine months before pregnancy. The third best time is at the start of pregnancy.

An amazing book that deals with effective preparation for pregnancy, among many other pertinent subjects, shows how far ahead of us—the supposed sophisticates—are many primitive cultures.

The book? *Nutrition and Physical Degeneration* was written by Dr. Weston Price, a Cleveland dentist who traveled around the world observing, interviewing, and photographing natives of primitive cultures. Don't be turned off by the fact that the book has been around for almost two generations. It's so old that it's new.[1]

Dr. Price compared the super-healthy natives in isolated areas of their land who thrive on native foods with those exposed to the fractional foods of modern civilization.

Actually the comparison was a *contrast*. Refined sugar and flour and other processed food had started causing rampant tooth decay and signs of every one of our degenerative diseases.

How to Raise Your Child's I.Q.—Part One 165

In our modern civilization, we emphasize the woman's need to prepare for pregnancy while overlooking the man's need to do the same. We can learn from some primitive cultures which, by custom, place both mothers-to-be and the fathers-to-be on special diets to assure their peak of health before they attempt conception.

Among Eskimos of the Arctic circle, for example, Dr. Price found that childbearing women prepared for pregnancy by eating fish eggs and fathers-to-be consumed milt, the sperm-containing fluid of salmon, to assure the highest degree of fertility and the liveliest sperm cells. During pregnancy as well the women ate a highly nutritious diet.

In the same regard, among Indians of the far north, both potential father and mother reinforce their health by eating organs of hunted wild animals.

Blueprint for Better Babies

Indicating that we have much to learn about developing better babies, Dr. Price describes how some cultures emphasize health-building diets long before planned pregnancies

Primitive peoples follow programs that will produce physically excellent babies—a simple but essential system of carefully planned nutritional programs for mothers-to-be. They begin this special feeding long before conception, not leaving it until after the mother-to-be knows she is pregnant.

Here are additional findings by Dr. Price:

Within the tradition of the primitive Masai in certain areas of Africa, young women were required to wait for marriage until the time of year when cows graze on young, green grass, and they can drink milk from these cows for a certain number of months.

In some agricultural African tribes, the young women are fed special foods for six months before marriage. In Fiji Dr. Price was shown a species of spider crab that the natives use for feeding mothers-to-be "so that their children will be physically excellent and mentally bright."

Natives of one South Pacific culture have a special tradition for the new mother. The young woman is required to tell the chief that she is pregnant. Promptly the chief arranges a collective feast to celebrate the "new person" who will soon join the colony.

Part of the ceremony involves the tribe's social security program. Members pledge themselves to adopt and care for the child if its parents die. During the feast, the chief appoints one or two young men to be responsible for bringing the pregnant woman special seafood needed to give her and the fetus the most nourishing fare available.

Upgraded Diet Before, During, and After Pregnancy

Many African tribes shared with Dr. Price that they had special foods for women to eat before pregnancy, during pregnancy, and during nursing. Throughout the nursing period, the mother was given red millet or linga-linga: two kinds of rich-in-nutrients cereal.

Upon analysis red millet was found to contain five to ten times the calcium of other cereals as well as other key vitamins and minerals. Of course, the natives knew nothing about calcium, only that the cereal helped to produce healthy, intelligent babies.

Linga-linga was also found to be highly nutritious. In fact, it is identical to quinoa (pronounced KEEN-wa) used in modern health cereals. High in trace mineral content, this grain stimulates the production and flow of breast milk. It has been used for this purpose by Peruvian Indians since the time of the Incas.[2]

Folk wisdom taught natives of these various cultures that mothers not only had to be in prime health to have babies, but also to produce top quality milk for breast-feeding infants. It taught them something more, according to Dr. Price: They should nurse the baby until he or she begins erupting teeth—no less than six months.

Better Than the Bottle

Countless research has verified the physical benefits of breast-feeding infants. Two key studies from the prestigious British medical journal *Lancet*, however, show that it boosts infants' I.Q. as well. The correlation held even when adjustments were made relative to the mothers' education and social class. Another significant finding: the more breast milk the child drinks, the higher the I.Q. in later life.

In the other study, 135 nine-year-olds who had been breast fed were compared with 391 nine-year-olds who had been bottle fed. Formula-fed children were twice as likely to have a neurological dysfunction. Such dysfunctions can often cause learning and behavioral difficulties.

Still another study, cited in a brochure by the Martek Corporation, makers of nutritional supplements, indicates that the Omega–3 fatty acid docosahexaenoic acid (DHA), a key component in breast milk, revved up the intelligence levels of more than 1,000 children. These children showed significant improvement in academic outcomes at several stages over an 18-year period.

A hazard in childbearing is the fact that some mothers are on reducing diets just before pregnancy, avoiding foods containing liberal amounts of fat—eggs, meat, organ meats, and cold-water fish. As a result, they also avoid a healthful intake of DHA. DHA is virtually absent from the diet of strict vegetarians

And many fail to take fish oil capsules of Omega–3 containing DHA and eicosapentaenoic acid (EPA) of flax oil capsules. This could be a serious mistake. As the mother deprives herself of DHA, she also deprives the breast-feeding baby. Numerous researchers have found that low levels of

DHA are linked to reduced ability to concentrate, memory loss, changes in disposition—usually negative—as well as neurological and visual disorders.

There is more DHA in the human brain than any other unsaturated fatty acid. It is the primary structural fat in both the brain's grey matter and the retina of the eye.

The *Feed Your Head* brochure, emphasizing the need for pregnant and nursing women to take in sufficient DHA, stresses the fact that

> Significant brain and eye development takes place in utero and continues during the first year after birth.
>
> Infants rely on their mothers to supply DHA for the developing brain and eyes initially through the placenta and then through breast milk. But, the average DHA level in the breast milk of American women is among the lowest in the world.

The brochure continues to the effect that during the late fetal stages and immediately following birth, the human brain grows very rapidly. "The DHA content of the fetal brain increases three to five times during the final trimester of pregnancy and triples yet again during the first 12 weeks of life."

Aside from the fact that breast milk of American women is now among the lowest in the world nutritionally speaking is this fact:

> The level of DHA in the mother's blood is depleted and takes time to return to pre-pregnancy levels [after birth].
>
> Premature babies are especially at risk for DHA deficiency, as are infants who are not breast fed, due to the fact that the U.S. infant formula is not enriched with DHA. One study has shown that the I.Q.s of

formula-fed infants are eight points lower, on average, than those of breast-fed babies.

More compelling information from *Feed Your Head* states that

the development of both the retina and visual cortex are similarly dependent on DHA. The retina develops rapidly during the final months of pregnancy and the first six months of infancy. One study found that the eyesight of full-term babies fed DHA-enriched formula was measurably more acute than that of babies fed formula without DHA. The difference in vision was equivalent to one line on an eye chart.

These are among the reasons an expert panel of the World Health Organization has recommended that all infant formula be enriched with DHA, as it is in 24 countries around the world.

A company named Martek Biosciences has created Neuromins™, a supplementary source of DHA from microalgae, the fish DHA source. Therefore, the supplement is right for meat-eaters *and* vegetarians.

Neuromins™ are distributed in retail outlets worldwide by major nutritional supplement companies such as Nature's Way, Neutraceutical Solaray® brand, Solgar Vitamin and Herb Company, and Source Naturals, Inc. Leiner Health Products markets Neuromins™ under its Your Life® label to more than 52,000 chain drug, supermarket, discount, and convenience retail stores in 50 states. The Neuromins product line is also available by phoning the manufacturer, Martek Biosciences Corporation at toll-free 1–800–662–6339.

DHA products of this firm come in three formulations: a 100 softgel capsule sold under the Neuromins DHA brand name, two 200 DHA softgel capsules Neuromins 200, and a product specifically formulated for pregnant and lactating women called Nueromins PL.

Relating findings on DHA and those of Dr. Weston Price, a gynecologist-obstetrician friend, made a profound statement to me recently:

"If all the couples who want intelligent and healthy babies read the ancient history in the Price book, they could rewrite modern history."

True. Then he said that, for all its remarkable medical advances, the United States has a disgraceful record among industrial nations in preserving the lives of newborn babies, ranking a lowly twentieth. Then he repeated a quotation by a wise anonymous person:

"The only lesson history has taught us is that man has not yet learned anything from history."

The Story of Defective Sperm

Up until recently at least, if conception fails, the woman is usually suspect—sometimes, even blamed. The same doctor friend I just mentioned pointed this out by telling the story of a young couple that couldn't conceive.

"Not only do we want a healthy baby," they told him, "we want one with a high I.Q., the drive and energy to be successful, and a personality to match."

He agreed to help the couple, but it took all his powers to convince them that the husband's sperm cells should be checked.

What the doctor saw through a high-powered microscope confirmed his hunch. Healthy sperm cells have a small, oval-shaped head and a stringlike appendage. As they swarm about, they are also driven forward with the vigorous screw-like action of their stringy tails. Few, if any, abnormally shaped cells should be present.

There was a contrasting picture on the slides. Sperm cells

were scarce, figuratively miles apart and some were oddly shaped, even with two heads. Others were too large or too small. Others still had two tails, one that split off from the cell below the head, like the straw of a broom sliced down the center.

Instead of moving vigorously, they moved slowly in labored confusion, as if they had forgotten or had never known their role in the pregnancy process. My doctor friend told the couple that sperm cells must have powerful thrust to propel themselves through the cervix, the uterus, and up five more inches to fertilize an egg.

Now this seems like a short trip. In comparison with their size, however, it is a long and arduous journey.

The story has a happy ending. The young man, a sedentary worker, promised to start a program of daily walking for exercise and to do everything else to make his and his wife's dream possible. His wife promised to do the same.

This commitment meant giving up their two to three cocktails nightly. They also eliminated candies and pastries, refined sugar and flour, and processed cereals and agreed to follow the diet the doctor designed for them.

Diet for Conceiving a Healthy, Brainy Baby

Diets for conceiving a healthy, brainy baby are very important. In fact, each meal should feature at least one fresh fruit or vegetable to furnish live enzymes which both aid in breaking down complex food molecules in preparing them for complete absorption. Processed foods cannot supply enzymes or the raw materials for the body to make them. That's why we need fresh plant foods. Any vegetable or food cooked at temperatures over 118°F loses its enzymes.

Please also note the structure of each meal. A high protein breakfast offers sustained energy. Dinners are purposely light. You don't need a heavy meal for watching TV and then sleeping. Milk is also mentioned in the diet. Many individuals though are milk-sensitive—secreting too little of the enzyme lactase to process lactose milk sugar, and suffering indigestion and other unpleasantness as a result. Some are also milk-allergic and suffer indigestion or flatulence (often both) and stomach pains, watering eyes, a snuffy nose, and frequent sneezing.

Nuts, however, are a major milk substitute, and those with the highest calcium content are almonds, pistachios, or walnuts. You can blend a half cup of these nuts with spring water, enough to cover the blender blades, plus a heaping tablespoon of carob powder to add natural sweetening, a delightful flavor, and 230 milligrams of calcium per 100 grams. It's quite a delicious drink!

If you feel, like some authorities, that there's no substitute for milk, try to buy the raw certified kind—it undergoes the most rigid inspection of any milk. If raw certified milk isn't available, there are some good low-fat products with added vitamin D. Homogenized milk has been indicted by one group of experts as a causative for heart attacks. Lactase-added milks are helpful to lactose-intolerant individuals. There are also brands of milk that are strictly organic. Cows are fed organic foods—no pesticides—and are not given antibiotics.

Here's the 7-Day Diet:

FIRST DAY

Breakfast

Whole wheat bagel and light cream cheese
Ground beef patty, 4 oz., broiled
Smoothie (fresh fruits: apple, peach, kiwi, banana, low-fat
  yogurt with lactobacillus acidophilus and other live
  cultures
Coffee substitute

Mid-Morning Snack

Muffin, buckwheat or bran

Lunch

Lentil soup, bowl
2 slices whole wheat toast, lightly buttered
Green salad, romaine lettuce—all you can eat—drizzled with flaxseed oil dressing—it contains DHA—and a hint of iodized salt
Milk, two percent fat or Nutty-Carob drink substitute

Mid-Afternoon Snack

Sunflower seeds, unsalted, 1 oz.

Dinner

Halibut, 4 oz., broiled
Irish potato, baked, served with pat of butter
Cabbage-carrot salad, grated, unsweetened yogurt dressing
Nutty-Carob drink (milk substitute)

SECOND DAY

Breakfast

2 eggs any style
Toast, two slices whole grain rye or wheat, lightly buttered (option: flaxseed oil spread)
Orange, Valencia, medium size
Coffee substitute, freshly brewed

Mid-Morning Snack

Popcorn, air-popped or lightly buttered, 1 cup

Lunch

Chicken soup, bowl
Whole grain crackers
Green salad: Romaine lettuce, alfalfa sprouts, olive oil
   dressing
Watermelon, ½ slice, 10″ × 1″ round
Spring water

Mid-Afternoon snack

Pecans, 10–12 halves

Dinner

Green pepper strips, 8–10
Small lamb chop, broiled
Irish potato, baked in skin, lightly buttered, sprinkled with
   dill and lightly seasoned with iodized salt
Strawberries, fresh, 14 medium, seven large with low-fat
   sour cream
Spring water

THIRD DAY

Breakfast

2 slices French Toast made with egg-milk (or egg and
   Nutty-Carob milk) batter, with wheat germ, cinnamon,
   vanilla. Maple syrup
Pear, fresh
Coffee substitute, freshly brewed

Mid-Morning Snack

Pumpkin seeds, unsalted, 1 oz.

Lunch

Beef broth (vegetarians: lentil soup)
Cheddar cheese toast, whole grain, 2 slices

Jicama slices, 8–10
Carrot sticks
Spring water

Mid-Afternoon Snack

Celery stalk, filled with macadamia butter

Dinner

Green salad, butter lettuce, all you can eat, soy dressing with a touch of iodized salt
Chicken, baked, 4 oz.
Apricots, 3 fresh
Spring water

FOURTH DAY

Breakfast

Cube steak, 4 oz.
Muffin, oat bran
Cantaloupe, half
Coffee substitute, freshly brewed or herbal tea

Mid-Morning Snack

Almonds, unsalted 8–10

Lunch

Tuna salad with Boston lettuce or other dark green, 3 oz. with sunflower seed oil dressing
Tangerine, medium
Herbal tea

Mid-Afternoon Snack

Pecans, 10 whole

Dinner

Chicken breast, 4 oz.
Brown rice, short grain, 1 cup, cooked and flavored with beef broth
Red raspberries, fresh, unsweetened, 1 cup
Milk, low-fat, or Nutty-Carob drink, 1 glass

FIFTH DAY

Breakfast

Whole orange
Creamed turkey on toast
Muffin, whole wheat with bran
Grapes, seedless, one cup
Coffee substitute, freshly brewed

Mid-Morning Snack

Walnuts, 10–12 halves

Lunch

Halibut, 4 oz., broiled
Asparagus spears, steamed, 6–8
Apple, winesap or green (Granny Smith)
Spring water

Mid-Afternoon Snack

Pecans, 1 oz.

Dinner

Caesar salad, large, with anchovies, blue cheese
Slice whole wheat pizza, heavy on tomato sauce, cheddar cheese, pumpkin seeds

Kiwi fruit, whole
Chamomile tea

DAYS SIX AND SEVEN

Repeat Days One and Two.

Importance of Essential Fatty Acids

The doctor put both the wife and husband on a daily vitamin B–complex tablet with major B–fractions of 50 milligrams and a multipurpose vitamin-mineral formula. (The husband's good health is of vast importance.) A key nutrient that they were also required to take—something that can't be included in multivitamin-mineral formulas—is essential fatty acids.

They are called "essential," for two reasons: Your body can't make them, and you have to have them. The doctor had them take 500 milligrams of Omega–3 and 1,000 milligrams of Evening Primrose Oil capsules daily. (The latter oils are the precursors of prostaglandins, entities that exercise short-term control of metabolism and every other major body function. They are also a part of cell membranes.) In addition the young man was asked to take three 500 milligram vitamin C tablets daily, one after each meal. Several studies show that this regimen contributes to male health and fertility.

Four months later, the doctor checked on the young man's sperm cells. This time they were plentiful, perfectly shaped, and in vigorous swarms. He was also pleased with the healthier physical appearance of the couple.

He suggested that they try again for pregnancy. They did. The happy ending was an eight-pound, two-ounce girl in radiant health.

The first secret to having a healthy and intelligent baby is to omit health-sabotaging lifestyle factors and add more healthy ones.

Healthy Baby "No-Nos"

As far as the health and welfare of the mother and baby-to-be are concerned, alcohol, tobacco and an inordinate amount of caffeine—as well as all drugs—should be eliminated whenever possible.

Alcohol shuts down the production of hydrochloric acid in the stomach, causing poor digestion and absorption of food, and, over a nine months' pregnancy, possible undernutrition.

Dozens of medical reports fail to offer any information as to whether or not it's safe to have even one alcoholic drink daily during pregnancy—partly because of our individual genetic differences and tolerances. So do your best not to drink during pregnancy. The risk is too great.

A Disastrous Procedure

Thankfully, the medical practice of administering alcohol to prevent premature birth has largely been abandoned. Several studies show this to be a mistake. Alcohol quickly enters the bloodstream. The concentration of alcohol in the mother's bloodstream and fetus is the same. If a premature birth should occur, a fetus with high levels of alcohol would have trouble surviving.

It is a physiological fact of life that in women and men of the same size drinking an equal amount of liquor, more alcohol ends up in the woman's bloodstream than in the man's.[3]

Why the difference? Charles Lieber, director of alcohol research and treatment at the Veterans Affairs Medical Center in New York City, theorizes that the difference arises in the stomach. There gender-related factors apparently accelerate the activity of alcohol-degrading enzymes. It's not fair, but women develop alcohol-related illnesses faster than men.

"We usually recommend that people drink moderately," Lieber states. However, his research suggests that clinicians should redefine "moderate" alcohol consumption for a very good reason. What's moderate for a man is not moderate for women or for people taking drug prescriptions.

Pregnancy already makes it necessary to take in a greater amount of vitamin B-1 than usual for metabolizing glucose for energy in our individual cells. Alcohol, a pure carbohydrate, like refined sugar and flour, demands its share of vitamin B-1.

Remember earlier, while talking about CATS—coffee, alcohol, tobacco, and sugar—we mentioned the idea of adding thiamin to alcohol to reduce serious consequences of alcohol drinking. In pregnancy, alcohol takes away a share of available vitamin B-1 and also interferes with the proper digestion of food, depriving mother and fetus of vitally necessary nutrients.

Alcohol Versus the B Vitamins

Other members of the vitamin B family depleted by excessive alcohol are B-2, B-6, niacin, and B-12. Vitamin B-2 is important for generating energy and protecting mucus membranes. Niacin, vitamin B-3, is also required for metabolizing alcohol.

Alcohol reduces the metabolism of vitamin B-6, a *must* for the brain and body to utilize essential amino acids, some of which end up as neurotransmitters, communicators between brain cells. It also stimulates the wasteful loss of this vitamin in the urine. Likewise, alcohol causes too great a loss of needed folic acid in the urine, a vitamin critical for ensuring normal cell division and repair, for making red blood cells, and for preventing deformities in the fetus: cleft palate, club feet, and spina bifida.

Alcohol diverts vitamin B-12 from entering the bones for forming red blood cells, for synthesizing DNA (the pattern for cell replication), for cell replicating, for preventing anemia, and for normal nervous system functioning essential for thinking and remembering. Added to all of this, alcohol also decreases the body's ability to absorb vitamin B-12.

In addition to its inordinate use and abuse of the entire vitamin B-complex, alcohol also takes its toll of vitamins C, D—a smaller amount of vitamin E—and the critically needed minerals: calcium, magnesium, manganese, zinc, chromium, copper, iodine, iron, and molybdenum. Alcohol is a known thief of many nutrients; so, it should not be permitted to gain access to the mother-to-be or her unborn child.

Author Dr. Roger J. Williams offers a way for alcoholics to break the habit: two to four grams of L-glutamine daily.[4] It is best to ingest this nutrient from supplements, inasmuch as it would take 10 grams of a high quality protein powder to offer one gram of L-glutamine.

How Tobacco Does Its Damage

Tobacco has unique ways of sabotaging the health of the mother-to-be and the fetus and interfering with a successful pregnancy.

Tobacco steals nutrients—particularly vitamin C, which is usually not storable in the human body for more than eight hours. Various experiments show that smoking one cigarette can remove 25 milligrams from the system. Vitamin C accelerates wound healing, boosts the immune system, helps with absorption of iron and calcium, contributes to solid bone formation, and protects against toxins.

Cigarettes depress appetite, making the pregnant woman less inclined to eat sufficient food, including nutrients that are a must for the fetus. Babies from smoking mothers are usually underweight and more subject to respiratory illnesses and allergies than infants from nonsmoking mothers.

Smoking narrows arteries, decreasing the flow of oxygen-bearing red blood cells to the fetus. Nicotine is also harmful to the fetus, as is the carbon monoxide in the smoke. It is the latter that decreases the amount of life-giving oxygen delivered to the baby, resulting in oxygen poverty.

If a mother seeks to preserve her health and that of her fetus, then she should stop drinking and smoking. Abstinence here protects against losing the baby or of the lesser but still traumatic possibility of having an infant handicapped physically or mentally.

Yes, stopping the nicotine habit is difficult, but it is not impossible. The best way to quit, of course, is never to have started. There are all sorts of props on the market to help kick the cigarette habit—nicotine gum and patches included. They all work for some people. I have known several patients who were able to quit smoking and drinking cold in order to have a healthy, intelligent baby. After the agony of resisting temptation throughout the pregnancy, they were able to quit for good, knowing that a child needs good air in the home for growing up in health and high intelligence.

Unfortunately, there is no quick solution for a habit that's easy to start and hard to quit, whether it be smoking or drinking. Still the Roger Williams' treatment for alcoholism—two to four grams of L-glutamine daily—has helped many people to quit, including a number of my patients.

CHAPTER 13

How to Raise Your Child's I.Q.—Part Two

Some years ago, a Welsh psychology professor innocently started a stampede to pharmacies and health food stores throughout Great Britain and, at the same time, unleashed the hostility of the medical establishment. All David Benton did was announce results of his study of 90 high school teenagers in an article in the prestigious British medical journal *Lancet*.[1]

Benton tested the students at the beginning and end of the school year. During the eight months in between, one-third of the group took a multivitamin and multimineral supplement. One-third received look-alike placebos, and the remaining one-third took nothing.

Result?

The supplemented students scored significantly higher in nonverbal I.Q. tests. Benton says that nonverbal I.Q. is a "more innate biological measure than verbal I.Q.," which is based more on formal learning and language. In addition, he felt that upgraded nutrition would be expected to influence nonverbal results prior to the verbal kind.

A BBC broadcast quoted the *Lancet* story in detail, and then everything hit the fan. Mired in the myth that "all anybody needs to stay healthy is a well-balanced diet," the medical establishment flogged Benton in the press.

How dare he attack typical British food? Why wasn't his study properly structured? How could he come to his conclusion with such a small sampling?

And the beat went on.

However, parents throughout Britain crowded health food stores and pharmacies for vitamins and minerals, as if these supplements were free.

An article on this subject in the *San Francisco Chronicle* expressed some skepticism about Benton's results with the sweeping statement: "It's a plausible theory. Though few children in the United States and Britain have marked nutritional deficiencies, many do have diets that are relatively low in iron and zinc, both of which are important to brain cell production.

"A recent study also implicated zinc deficiency as a risk factor in dyslexia," the article continued. "The B vitamins, also low in some kids' diets, support brain function, too."

Better Diet, Better Grades

About the same time, another article on a similar subject appeared in newspapers across the nation and raised eyebrows in the educational and orthodox medical communities.

Fortunately for us, the 'Doubting Thomases' began to lose some of their doubt. A three-year study by Stephen Schoenthaler, Ph.D., Walter Doraz, and James Wakefield, Jr., of California State University, Stanislaus, presented strong evidence that an enhanced diet can contribute to higher school grades.[2]

No one could protest that the sampling was too small. Academic levels of one million New York City public elementary and junior high school students were evaluated periodically, before and after school lunches were enhanced. They showed improvement.

Dramatic rises in scores surprised school officials, if not

the researchers. Average test scores of 803 New York City schools rose by 15 percent within four years after the school lunch program was upgraded.

New York City's public schools rated in the thirty-ninth percentile in 1979, as shown by the standardized California Achievement Test scores used nationwide, indicating that 61 percent of the nation's other school systems scored higher.

Then in 1980, the New York City Board of Education reduced the sugar content of foods and banned two artificial food colorings in school lunches. Later that year, achievement test scores rose markedly—this time to the forty-seventh percentile nationwide.

Impressed by what was happening, New York City public school officials outlawed foods with artifical coloring and flavoring. Once more, test scores rose—this time to the fifty-first percentile.

Next, foods containing two common preservatives, BHT and BHA, were removed from the school lunch. Again, scores of city schools rose—now to the fifty-fourth percentile. How much this was due to the change in diet is perhaps arguable. But the change itself spoke volumes and did wonders for the schools and their students.

More Evidence

Junk foods were banned. Milk replaced carbonated beverages and candy. And New York schools achieved something beyond a 15 percentile academic gain, overwhelming as that was. They realized a tremendous cost saving. The schools required fewer special education teachers to offer individual instruction to children with reading problems, indicated Doraz.

The study by Schoenthaler and associates is especially significant because it spotlights typical mind-body saboteurs in the American diet: excessive sugar and artificial additives, including food colorings—many derived from coal tar and, therefore, carcinogenic—emulsifiers and preservatives.

Although this study is admirable on its own terms, there are many more factors to consider about American food and its influences on the minds of the young—on those of any age group, for that matter. These start from the ground up.

The late William A. Albrecht, Ph.D., while chairman of the Department of Soils at the University of Missouri, discovered through many studies that declining soil fertility is reducing the ability of crops to synthesize protein.[3] (This is something for strict vegetarians to consider.)

Within a ten-year period, protein content of corn decreased from 9.5 to 8.5 percent. Certain amino acids normally present—components of protein—disappeared entirely. Carbohydrate content increased as soils became more depleted of trace minerals.

"The same thing is happening to our wheat," Albrecht stated, reminding us that we are at the top of the biotic pyramid, supported by and as dependent on a base of animals, plants, microbes, and soil, as they are dependent upon us. If this base fails, so do we. The answer: Eat more organically grown foods from a rapidly increasing number of organic farmers.

The mass switch to hybrid seeds by agribusiness—farmers no more—is producing crops with a lower nutrient content. Then too, many seeds are treated with pesticides before being planted.

Problems From the Ground Up

Today's agricultural practices cause soil to become mineral-poor through erosion, nonrotation of crops, and synthetic fertilizers that replace only a small fraction of trace minerals taken out by crops. The fertilizers leave behind nitrates that end up in our food and water supply.

Toxic fungicides, herbicides, and insecticides on foods are another hazard. Most fruits and vegetables are picked when immature, before they have time to ripen to the full potential of their food values. Then they are artificially ripened.

Factory farming contrasts sharply with grazing cattle on the open range. Two artificial devices are used to make cattle gain weight and bring higher profits: hormones and crowded feedlots (standing room only). Close quarters cause the spread of disease and, therefore, the need for antibiotics.

Magic doesn't make the hormones and antibiotics disappear entirely. Some of it ends up in the meat and in us.

Chickens also live under artificial, even brutal conditions, packed together on stretches of wire mesh—not on the ground. Diseases spread easily and quickly and call for antibiotics, some of which remain in the meat.

Inasmuch as pesticides accumulate more in animals than plants, many people choose to be vegetarians, faced with an ever-declining protein intake.

Many water sources are polluted from industrial waste and pesticides, as well as from nitrate fertilizers washed into creeks, rivers, and lakes. A strong suspect as a cancer-causative, chlorine in water kills most of the microorganisms there, but it may take many years before we know what a number it's doing on us.

The Graduation of Rat Poison

As mentioned earlier, a genius at recycling came up with a great idea for getting rid of fluoride, the waste product of aluminum makers and producers of synthetic fertilizers: Protect children's teeth from caries (the fancy name for cavities) by fluoridating municipal water supplies.

One needs rubber statistics to stretch them far enough to show an advantage for the teeth of children in fluoridated communities compared with those in nonfluoridated communities.

Previously one of the better rat poisons and a well-known thyroid gland suppressant, fluoride was initially added to water supplies at just one part per million. Several years ago, the Environmental Protection Agency raised that to a range of from one to four parts per million. At the higher rate, companies will have to produce more aluminum and synthetic fertilizer to keep up with demand for fluoride.

Seriously, fluoride is now becoming an even more hazardous problem. It comes at us not only in water supplies but in products made in fluoridated water cities—soft drinks, beer, fruit juices, processed foods. This is in addition to that in toothpaste and mouthwashes. Thankfully, the FDA has finally made toothpaste manufacturers add a warning of toxicity to the labeling of fluoridated toothpastes.

Already touched upon lightly is the problem of fractionated foods, mainly white flour. So that flour would not spoil readily, could be shipped distances, and store well, millers removed the vitamin- and mineral-rich germ and outer husk. These nutritious parts were fed to hogs, and all other parts were reserved for us human beings.

Just as a toll bridge takes our money, heating, canning, drying, and freezing food costs us many nutrients. Food additives—colors, preservatives, emulsifiers—only introduce a Las Vegas element to eating.

Chemical Warfare Against Eaters

James Braly, M.D., states that there are "over 3,000 chemicals—that is, produced by a chemical process—added to the American diet every day."[4]

"It is now well established," he continues "that some of these chemicals actually have the ability to change the digestive process and distort the permeability of the intestinal lining, the last barrier between the outside world and your bloodstream."

Apologists tell us not to worry about added toxins. After all, fruits, vegetables, and grains all have their own in-built toxins, courtesy of Mother Nature. So then, do we need a double dip?

There's a newspaper article on the desk before me to the effect that about 100,000 people die from prescribed medicines each year. Of all places, the original version of that article appeared in the *Journal of the American Medical Association*.[5]

One point the article makes should give you pause: Some of these untimely deaths resulted from two medicines that, when taken together, become poisonous. What are our chances of survival—brain and all—with 3,000 chemical additives? We can be thankful that they're not all in the same foods.

Health author Barbara Kahan adds that foods most incriminated in children's learning and behavior problems are highly refined, highly sweetened, colored with food dyes, and preserved with BHA and BHT. Then too, there are foods contaminated with lead, mercury, and aluminum or containing caffeine, as well as sound foods, to which some children may be sensitive.[6]

What's the answer for survival so long as it's important for us to continue eating, drinking, and breathing?

Let's Ride the Wave of Change!

Organically grown foods, for one. They have been in health food stores for decades and now are quietly invading supermarkets. Raley's, a chain of supermarkets based in Sacramento, California, sells organically grown vegetables and fruits. It's the start of a trend. Your dollars and ours have power to convert other chains to organic foods. Let's make that money talk—to store managers!

Individuals whose parents or grandparents were active during World War II might have heard about Victory Gardens, backyard plots of ground where people grew their own vegetables and fruit to help the war effort. For somebody who has a decent size backyard, a Victory Garden for organically grown produce is an idea worth reviving.

So much for gaining positive advantages for body and brain by eliminating the negative. What are some of the positive things that can be done?

Invariably, when I appear on radio or TV talk shows or when I lecture, concerned mothers tell me they want an easy way to upgrade their children's diet. If I mention a book of recipes, they turn off.

"Most recipe books—even the best ones for organic cookery—offer complicated recipes that call for ingredients I don't keep on hand. Who needs to go ingredient hunting. Time is precious. I want something simple."

A Simple Way to Win

In these hurry-up days when there's too much to do in too little time, it's best to work from where you are. We live in a real world. Choose foods the kids like and add more nourishment to them, trying not to change the basic taste so much that it turns them off.

Most kids like hamburgers. You start with low-fat ground meat. (Fortunately, there's a growing number of outlets for organically raised, no pesticide, no hormone, no antibiotic meat. Check the Yellow Pages.) Organically grown beef costs a little more than supermarket meat, but, then it's more healthful. Let's face it. Doctors don't come cheap either.

Now that you have top quality ground beef, you beat an egg and blend it into the meat, along with a tablespoon of wheat germ. You broil it well so that the fat melts away, and you kill the possible *E. coli* organisms to prevent illness or death. Then you serve the hamburgers on whole wheat buns. As an alternative, ground turkey is available for hamburgers. So is buffalo burger in some areas.

For brain and body building, wheat germ is one of your best bets for making everyday foods more nutrition-dense. It's loaded with goodies. A half cup contains 24 grams of protein, about as much as a quarter pound of turkey, more than four ounces of ground beef, and four times as much as an egg.

Remember the Ruth Flinn Harrell experiment and how vitamin B–1 helped to boost the I.Q.s of kids from five to 87 percent? Well, a half cup of wheat germ contains 2½ milligrams of B–1, almost a day's supply, according to the U.S. government's Recommended Daily Allowance (RDA). Wheat germ is also one of the richest foods in other B vitamins—vitamin B–2, niacin, vitamin B–6, pantothenic acid, and inositol.

Its abundant vitamin E, a powerhouse antioxidant, helps to process unsaturated fatty acids—important to brain health and activity.

Wheat germ is super-rich in trace minerals closely related to high brain function: copper, magnesium, manganese, and potassium. It is also rich in phosphorus, one of the brain's favorite minerals. Only there's a small problem here. It lacks calcium. Unless calcium comes from another source, phosphorus may be dominant and draw residual calcium out of the body with it.

Milk helps to compensate for this, but has drawbacks for some individuals. Soy milk, available everywhere, is a good, though not complete, substitute for cow's milk. Nonetheless it is near the top of the list of calcium-rich foods.

Wheat germ deteriorates quickly, so buy it in small

amounts and keep it tightly closed and in the refrigerator when not in use.

Nutty Way to Better Nutrition

One thing I always impress upon mothers is to buy the best grade of peanut butter, a product that contains no hydrogenated oil, sugar, preservatives, or other additives. (Peanut butter is such a favorite food of children that it pays to go first class.) Makers of this product still do not guarantee peanuts free of the carcinogenic aflatoxin mold. However, if we continue to request that store managers urge their chief executives to pressure peanut butter makers to offer an untainted product, we will soon get one. We also must bombard peanut butter processors with the same forceful requests.

Nutrition centers carry nut spreads that are not hydrogenated and loaded with preservatives. Slowly, supermarkets are beginning to sell such products, too. Various national chain stores and gourmet food stores feature a variety of nut butters: cashew, almond, and macadamia, products not as likely to be subject to aflatoxin mold.

Certain mothers make the error of substituting margarine for butter in these times of fanaticism against saturated fats. This is sad, because they are gaining nothing and losing something. To turn an oil into a solid such as margarine, it must be at least partially hydrogenated, a process that converts the healthful "cis" form of fat to "trans" fats, actual antinutrients that prevent development of prostaglandins, hormone-like substances, short-term regulators of the central nervous system, cardiovascular system, reproductive system, and the immune system.

One of the best books on essential fatty acids, *The Nutrition Superbook: The Good Fats and Oils,* edited by Jean Barilla, states:

"Some researchers believe that the onset of any disease

can be attributed to prostaglandin imbalance. Research continues to show that margarine clogs arteries as relentlessly as saturated fat does and is linked to tumor growth in animals.''

Butter, an excellent food, should be used in moderation, except by individuals afflicted with a rare inherited medical condition, familial hypercholesterolemia, extremely high blood cholesterol. As a butter substitute, some mothers offer virgin olive oil as a dip for bread.

Most kids like pizza, so this Italian import offers lots of possibilities for creative and nutritious additions. One of my patients, the mother of two kids created a plan through which she could build her own healthful ingredients into pizza. She announced a new game to the kids. She would bake the crust—naturally out of whole wheat flour—and on different evenings her young son and slightly older daughter would each be able to include whatever ingredients they wished.

One of the rules established was that all members had to agree to eat each other's pizza. (Many health food stores carry ready-mixed whole wheat pizza crusts for busy mothers.)

That worked fine until the young boy topped the tomato sauce and grated cheese pizza with marshmallows!

How About That Tomato!

Marshmallows aren't considered to be a health food, *but tomatoes are.* The last three words should be written in flaming letters. They are that important. Everyone who cooks for him- or herself or others should know that the red coloring substance in tomatoes is the incredible antioxidant lycopene, mentioned briefly at the end of the chapter on Alzheimer's disease. Jim Scheer and I consider lycopene the crown jewel of nutrients.

Many of us in preventive health are zealous about preaching the merits of raw vegetables and fruit. And this is certainly justified from the standpoint of their live enzymes and fiber, as well as nutrients that are diminished by cooking.

Cooking, however, causes no harm to the lycopene in tomatoes. In fact, cooking seems to make lycopene more assimilable. Biochemist John W. Erdman, Ph.D., at the University of Illinois at Chicago, has researched lycopene for decades and, in many public statements, tells us that it is fat soluble and best absorbed when accompanied by some fat, as in processed tomato products. Like what? Like tomato sauce, tomato paste, spaghetti sauce, and ketchup.

"A salad with tomatoes and a fat-free salad dressing won't do it," states Dr. Erdman. "Stick to low-fat dressings, or eat the salad with other foods that contain fats."

Early research on benefits of lycopene failed to get through to the eating public. It was esoteric writing: long words and biochemical jargon. Then came the breakthrough, a paper published in the December 1995 issue of the *Journal of the National Cancer Institute.*

Written by Edward Giovannucci, M.D., and colleagues at the Harvard University School of Public Health, the paper revealed in plain English results of a six-year, epidemiological study of 47,000 men. Those who ate 10 or more servings of tomato-based foods each week were 45 percent less likely to develop prostate cancer.

Since then, numerous studies show that, as an antioxidant, lycopene is a giant killer, able to quench one of the most vicious free radicals to attack brain and body cells, the singlet oxygen free radical. The singlet oxygen radical damages walls of cells in brain and body, as well as their DNA, undermines enzymes so they can't perform their work, denatures or destroys protein, and weakens the immune function.

Lycopene is one of the most staunch defenders of brain and body cells—more potent than the powerful carotenoid, beta carotene. Many studies demonstrate that it seems to interfere with cancer cell growth and spread and blocks the development of rapidly growing cancer cells more effectively than other carotenoids—beta and alpha carotene, among them.

Animal and human research suggests that it may suppress breast tumors, decrease the risk of devastating pancreas cancer, lung cancer, and cancers of the digestive tract, mouth, esophagus, stomach, colon, and rectum. Further, it appears to guard against cardiovascular disease. It protects smokers. Epidemiological studies indicate that smokers with low blood levels of lycopene have three times the risk of cancer than those with high levels.

Lycopene is such an important nutrient that I urge patients to eat cooked tomato products in meals at least three times weekly—for themselves and their children.

For patients so busy that they can't always include enough tomato products in their menus, I recommend a lycopene supplement—one to two capsules daily. The best lycopene product I know (Lyc-O-Mato™) is made by Lyco Red Natural Products Industries, of Beer-Shiva, Israel, and sold to major nutritional supplement companies that distribute it under their own labels through health food stores. Ask your health food store manager or clerk to guide you to the right product.

Lyc-O-Mato is different in that it is based on unique tomatoes—none like them anywhere else in the world. These tomatoes were developed by special plant agro-breeding techniques that produce luscious, vine-ripened tomatoes which contain three times more lycopene than ordinary tomatoes. *No genetic engineering* was involved.

Lycopene is extracted *without commonly used chemicals* that leave a residue. When you buy a lycopene supplement, be sure you get one based on Lyc-O-Mato from Lyco Red Natural Product Industries.

This lycopene coverage may have seemed to be a lengthy excursion away from the subject of nutrition-dense meals prepared at home. However, it was too important to omit or deal with in just a handful of wisely selected words.

Creative Upgrading of Nutrition

Desiccated liver contains the B–complex, the thinking person's vitamins, and also something that wheat germ doesn't have, vitamin B–12—one of the most important nutrients for retaining an excellent memory.

In a household I know well, a father and single parent upgraded his children's nutrition by means of one of their favorite foods: stuffed peppers. He enriched the ground meat stuffing for the peppers with a tablespoon of powdered, nutritious desiccated beef liver.

"This tastes a little different," Mary Ann, the pre-teen daughter remarked. "But it isn't bad."

Another way of inducing anemic or otherwise weak patients to take desiccated liver is to stir a level teaspoonful in a large glass of tomato juice. Even that small amount taken every three or four days helps build strength. After a few months of conditioning the kids to the taste, you can get away with adding a heaping teaspoonful to the juice.

Many times kids reject a food without even trying it. A creative mother asked her teenage son what he would like added to broiled beef liver. He requested garlic salt and fried onions. She complied. He ate it slowly, reluctantly, and, soon, with pleasure.

Seafood, and the old legend about being brain food attached to it, is very true. Fish is indeed brain food. The high concentration of Omega–3 oil in salmon and cold water fish like halibut, haddock, and cod makes them good fare for including in the diet several times a week.

An ingenious mother invented a game called "No Complaint" that made it possible for her to introduce and repeat nutrition-packed meals for her teenagers. Here is the rule of the game. If someone utters the least objection to the dish prepared by the mother, that kid has the job of buying the food and cooking it for the next night. It worked because, after the novelty of cooking wears off, the kids would rather just eat and be done with it. The mother was able to introduce many new super-nutritious dishes that were accepted without a murmur.

And Vitamins, Too

Of course, all of the mothers mentioned made a post-breakfast rule that the kids had to supplement this meal with multivitamins and multiminerals. Kids grow rebellious if they have to take a lot of individual vitamins, as many health-conscious adults do. Taking a few supplements regularly until the daily habit is ingrained is important though.

One of the best all-purpose supplements for kids up to 12 years of age is the animal-shaped, pleasant-tasting, chewable wafers called AMNI Kids®. All ingredients are chosen for purity, potency, and easy assimilability. This product meets U.S. pharmaceutical standards. Potencies listed on the label are exactly what you get.

There's a date stamp on the bottle to assure freshness of the product. AMNI Kids is free of artificial additives and contains 27 vitamins, minerals, and trace elements. Two wafers are to be taken daily, one with breakfast and another with lunch or dinner. Most health food stores carry AMNI Kids. If they don't they can order them for you by phoning 1-800-356-4791.

Breakfast

Breakfasts That Shatter Convention

Even the staid U.S. Department of Agriculture warns about serving the same foods for breakfast every day—cereal, for instance. There's nothing wrong with being

How to Raise Your Child's I.Q.—Part Two   197

unconventional. If your boy or girl likes chop suey, and you had some left from the night before, warm it up for breakfast. Don't hesitate to serve hamburgers for breakfast.

Pancakes are usually a favorite for kids. You can add eggs and wheat germ to the whole grain batter, along with bits of pecans or walnuts—whatever he or she likes—and serve a nutritious meal.

One mother I know adds carob, a highly nutritious chocolate substitute to hotcake batter. Carob is also called St. John's bread, because John the Baptist sustained himself in the desert by eating carob pods. It is high in vitamins—particularly vitamin B–1, the brain vitamin, essential for the proper digestion of carbohydrates, a positive spirit, and healthy nerves. It contains many trace minerals, including a balance of phosphorus and calcium. Carob is not only a rich-in-protein food, but it also contains built-in sweetening.

One mother was disappointed that her daughter thought carob "is not chocolaty enough," but it gave her an idea. She mixed some cocoa in with it, and then the carob-spiked hot cakes tasted chocolaty enough.

"You have to use all your wiles to get some kids to eat the things that are good for them," she told me. "You've got to be realistic and be pleased with small nutritional gains. Better a combination of carob and chocolate than all chocolate!"

A lot of mothers who are my patients use molds for making and freezing fresh fruit juice Popsicles as wholesome desserts. Also, some get the family involved in making ice cream at home. This way fresh fruits can be added, along with nuts.

Poor Breakfast, Low Energy

Above all else, it is critically important for everyone to eat a substantial breakfast. A few quick sips of coffee and an in-flight doughnut down the front steps aren't calculated to supply the energy and brain power for a morning in school or at work.

Studies have proved again and again that a good protein breakfast is a *must* for a day of major league brain work. However, one of the first and most impressive studies was done many years ago by E. Orent-Keiles and L.F. Hallman at the U.S. Department of Agriculture. We owe them, and the department a debt of gratitude.[7]

Various breakfasts were tested on 200 volunteers. Each one's blood sugar was checked before the meal and every hour for three hours afterward. Just a cup of black coffee caused the blood sugar to decrease accompanied by irritability, nervousness, hunger, fatigue, exhaustion, and headaches. These conditions worsened as the morning ground toward noon.

Coffee with sugar and cream and two doughnuts worked a little better. Blood sugar at least climbed for the first hour, then it dropped to a low level, bringing about fatigue and some of the same symptoms experienced with just the black coffee.

Next came what the researchers called a "Basic Breakfast," because it was typical of that eaten by millions of Americans: a glass of orange juice, two strips of bacon, toast, jam, and coffee with cream and sugar.

Up went the blood sugar for an hour and then it nosedived way lower than the prebreakfast level, staying there until lunch.

Foods of the next breakfast were identical to those of the previous one with one addition: a packaged cereal. The blood sugar stayed high for about an hour then dropped to the prebreakfast low.

For the next breakfast, cooked oatmeal with cream and sugar was added to the Basic Breakfast in place of the prepared cereal. Again, the blood sugar soared quickly but plummeted in less than an hour to a level lower than any of the previous ones measured.

Once more the Basic Breakfast of orange juice, bacon, toast, jam, and coffee was upgraded with another item: this time eight ounces of whole milk fortified by 2½ tablespooons of powdered milk. (For those who can't drink milk, a combination of carob, nuts, and spring water can be blended into a milk substitute.)

This meal brought the blood sugar level up to normal, where it stayed all morning. Volunteers on this fare felt high-spirited, happy, and mentally alert until noon.

In the next breakfast, two eggs were added to the Basic Breakfast, rather than the fortified milk. The blood sugar rose and stayed just as high as on the previous breakfast. Again, the volunteers experienced high energy, mental alertness, and a feeling of well-being until noon.

The last breakfast was similar to the previous one, except that more toast and jam were added to either eggs or fortified milk with the Basic Breakfast. Blood sugar rose high and stayed there.

High Protein Breakfast Proves Itself

What happened next proved that the breakfasts with a high level of protein—fortified milk or eggs—had a value far beyond merely sustaining the volunteers until noon.

Every one of the volunteers—from the person who had only black coffee to those who ate the Basic Breakfast plus eggs or fortified milk—was given the same lunch: a cream cheese sandwich on whole grain bread and a glass of whole milk.

In every case the blood sugar rose, but it was only a brief rise and then came a morale-lowering fall for those who didn't eat the Basic Breakfast plus either the eggs or fortified milk. And it stayed down the whole afternoon.

However, it was dramatically different for the Basic Breakfast people who ate the breakfast of high protein eggs or drank the whole fortified milk. These people reached a high blood sugar level that lasted them all afternoon.

This and other studies prove that a breakfast that generates a sustained high blood sugar level until noon helps to continue that high all afternoon even on a light lunch. Numerous studies have proved that a hearty high protein breakfast sustains students in a cheerful, positive, and I-can-handle-it attitude conducive to open-mindedness to learning, a good attention span necessary for taking in new information, and the ability to remember.

Who Says You Can't Eat Breakfast?

So many children, youths, and adults claim they can't eat a full breakfast. The nutrition authority Adelle Davis once told me there's a simple solution to that: have the person eat only a light dinner or none at all. After a while, an appetite for breakfast will develop.

Adelle's advice has worked for my patients. In general, those who have a clear-cut goal and a strong desire to reach it discipline themselves to eat a solid breakfast. Knowing they can sustain high energy all day, they also reverse their eating habits. They see quite clearly why they don't need to eat their heaviest meal at night simply to watch TV or read and then go to sleep. They know their heaviest meal should come in the morning when the greatest amount of energy and the highest morale are needed for a day at school or at work.

An added benefit of this reversal—the heaviest meal in the morning and the lightest in the evening—is that it helps those who want to lose weight. A study published in the *Journal of the Louisiana State Medical Society* stresses this point.[8]

On a solid foundation of nutrient-dense food and a good breakfast, a young person can build. A second step is to develop a physically fit body. Remember in Chapter 2, we showed how regular exercise stimulates the brain. Usually competitive games such as tennis work best for young people—better than just walking, a monumental bore for kids and youths. Swimming, skateboarding, surfing—any sustained and aerobic exercise done regularly—are excellent activities here as well.

A Modern Genius Shares His Secrets

The system for preparing the mind that is fundamentally sound was developed by Dr. Naka-Mats, of Japan, a world class inventor. This modern day genius who invented the floppy disk and licensed it to IBM—as well as the compact disc, the CD player, and the digital watch—has invented twice as many patented devices as Thomas Edison, a past American genius.

In several interviews Dr. Naka-Mats indicated that every sort of educational exposure for children is important. The Japanese system, for instance, stresses memorization for children and youths up to age 20. Then they have the basis for free association and creating new ideas.

But whether or not memorization is *the* educational tool in helping a child achieve, it is to the parents that much responsibility falls. A parent truly interested in the child's welfare and self-expression, for instance, should help the child discover his or her interests. This is the belief of Dr. Naka-Mats, who admitted how fortunate he was to have parents who encouraged his natural curiosity along with his academic learning from the start. "They gave me the freedom to create and invent, which I have been doing from the very beginning," he stated.[9]

Cultivating Creativity

There are many ways that parents can can help their children develop creativity. One is to play games, especially in figuring out other uses for common devices.

Take a metal pail for instance, and see how many different objects your child's imagination can make of it.

Turn it over, and it can be a seat. Fill it with dirt, and it can become a flower pot. Turn it over and put it on your head, and it is a hat. Place it on the hallway floor, and you have an umbrella stand. Turn it over again, and you can use it as a step stand. Fill it with water, and minnows can swim in it. Paint it different colors, hang it in the den, and it is a work of art. Well, you get the idea. Do the same with any common object, and encourage your child to do some mind-stretching.

Companies are always staging contests to get ideas for new uses for old products. Children get valuable creative experience by entering contests, even if they don't win a prize.

The "What if" game is a winner. It's also the game that Jim Scheer used when he wrote fiction. While in a zoo, he asked what would life be like if we were caged and the apes ran the world? (Maybe they have taken over!) What if people could live for 150 years? (The Social Security system doesn't need any more ideas about how to go broke.) What if the president, vice president, and the Speaker of the House were all kidnapped and no one could find them? What if rivers suddenly ran uphill? What if people, tired of high ticket prices, suddenly stopped attending athletic events?

This mind-stretcher is fun, because your kids and you can enjoy the creativity of constructing the whole plot for a novel or play. Be sure not to monopolize the "what-iffing."

Imagination is another fun game—especially on a sunny day when lots of clouds are scudding across the sky. Simply lie in the grass and look up. Let the clouds take you. And listen as your child tells you what he or she sees: a bear, a snowman, a horse, and so on.

Turn Their Imaginations Loose!

Encourage your child to ask questions. You won't know all the answers, but this will give you a chance to work together to find answers perhaps in a library or on the Internet.

Every time a local business or your fire station has an open house, try to take your child there and encourage him or her to ask questions. Every exposure will offer opportunities to learn about something new.

Another way to develop imagination is to select a room in the house—take the bathroom—and examine every product in it, including the fixtures and figure out how to improve them.

In one bathroom, a large mirror was held in place with a horizontal metal strip at the bottom. It was like a narrow gutter. Water splashed up, gathered there, and worked its way inside the glass, making unsightly, streaky, black patterns on the bottom.

A little girl noted this and asked, "Why don't they just hold the mirror in place with three little pieces of metal. That way no water would collect and spoil the looks of the mirror."

Common sense and creativity go hand-in-hand here. Guided to looking for ways to improve products in the house and the outside world, this small girl is on her way to becoming an inventor, even perhaps a world class one.

Encourage your kid to start a business and work with him or her as a consultant every step of the way. This would be something more original than a lemonade stand.

One kid wanted to start a Saturday and after-school delivery business with his new bike. He and his dad designed a sidecar for carrying things—a creative learning experience for both of them. It was made easily detachable so that the youngster could still ride the bike to school.

He designed some handbills to sell his service, took them to an instant printer, and then delivered them with a smile to the owner of every store that seemed a likely prospect. Convenience stores and drug stores turned out to be his best customers. Now he makes all of his spending money and is saving up for a used car when he's old enough to get a driver's license.

A young man in Pennsylvania saved his spending money and bought many distress sale athletic shoes that he sold at a profit in public parks and gyms. Every buy and sell taught him how to be more efficient. Ten years later he has learned where to find and sell distress sale merchandise of all kinds. He now owns a $25 million a year business.

Starting a business takes creativity to see a need, figure out how to fill it, and then take the initiative to approach and win customers.

Planning, funding, starting, and building a business exercises a kid's creativity, ingenuity, and business and social skills. It could be the training that develops a brilliant entrepreneur in your family!

And why not? In terms of creativity, the sky's the limit.

CHAPTER 14

The Summing Up

1. Making of a Genius

Professor Robert Rivera's physical exercises send the I.Q. skyrocketing—as much as 30 points! Remember the first exercise: Inhale for eight counts. Hold your breath for 12 counts, then slowly exhale for 10 counts. Repeat 10 times. Here's how to do Professor Rivera's second I.Q.-raising exercise: Flatten your back against the wall, then stretch upward. Do this 10 times. Some individuals feel that both exercises skyrocket their I.Q.s to the highest levels.

The rest of the chapter reveals many other ways of reaching your I.Q.'s peak potential.

2. Exercise the Brain for Better Thinking

When you solve problems or wrestle with mental challenges, the tree-like dendrites of your brain cells grow and microcirculation expands to bring more blood and oxygen to your brain to improve your thinking. Without challenges, dendrites and brain microcirculation shrink, and thinking becomes sluggish. Remember the good things that happened to Dr. Marian Diamond's challenged rats!

3. The Importance of Being Oxygenated

Keep oxygenated blood vigorously making the rounds through clean arteries with physical and mental exercises! Your brain uses oxygen, glucose, and a minute amount of thyroid hormone to develop energy for thinking. Too little thyroid hormone, hypothyroidism—often a hidden and, therefore, an undiagnosed condition in 40 percent of the population—causes low body temperature that slows thinking and remembering.

The no-cost, do-it-yourself Barnes Basal Temperature Test tells you the state of your thyroid gland. Thyroid supplementation can sometimes work wonders with your mind and body. It may be the exact factor you need to vault you into major league thinking, remembering, and career accomplishment.

4. Nutrients That Skyrocket Your I.Q.

Ginkgo biloba, an ancient Chinese herb that promotes better blood circulation, is essential to improving brainpower. In an incredible experiment by Elizabeth Flinn Harrell with another nutrient—vitamin B–1—raised the I.Q.s of children by from 7 to 87 percent. L-glutamine is another supplement that stimulates the brain for better and faster thinking. These and other supplements can make you a part of the brain trust!

5. Brain Transplant or Something Better?

Exotic nutritional supplements such as phosphatidylserine, acetyl-L-carnitine and DMAE give you better mileage from your brainpower. Phosphatidylserine has been called a "brain detergent," helpful in Parkinson's and Alzheimer's disease. Actetyl-L-carnitine powers fuel into brain cell "furnaces" to give you greater brain energy, clearer thinking, and a more dependable memory. In a test of task performance, DMAE enabled volunteers to master tests faster and with fewer errors than those who took placebos.

6. CATS and Your Mind

C-A-T-S—coffee, alcohol, tea and sugar—can undermine your health and mind. A cup of coffee is excellent for starting the metabolic motor in the morning. However, experts warn against drinking more than four cups daily. It depletes vitamin B-1 so critical in raising I.Q. Alcoholism can turn the brain into mush. Even moderate alcohol intakes can steal critically needed vitamin B-1. Tobacco is noted for shrinking arteries and limiting the flow of blood, oxygen, and nutrients to the brain. Innocent-looking sugar that tastes so good also is a vitamin B-1 thief. CATS, indeed, steal brain power. Habituation makes it so difficult to get rid of CATS that they seem to have nine lives!

7. Heavy Metals and Your Brain

Toxic metals—lead, aluminum, cadmium, and mercury—are decreasing our mentality. Our lead load is incredible. A study of 7- to 11-year-old boys shows that lead interferes with ability to pay attention (limiting learning), lowers I.Q.s, and promotes antisocial behavior. The Brain Bio Center discovered that 2,000 mg of vitamin C and 60 mg of zinc daily can draw lead out of the body. Chelation can reduce both the lead and cadmium load. Cadmium, of course, can cause mental retardation. Mercury intoxication makes thinking difficult and can cause memory loss. You, too, can learn how to rid yourself of these toxins and rev up your mental powers by the process of eliminating them.

8. Stress: The Mind-Killer

Stress burdens the heart *and* arteries. A dramatic study shows the sabotage it can do to body and brain. Arteries with moderate plaque narrowed by 9 percent under stress, and arteries with heavy plaque narrowed by 24 percent under stress. Smooth arteries expanded slightly. You know the major stressors in your life. However, there are subtle and hidden ones that are clouding your thinking, stealing your memory, and shortening your life. World authority Dr. Cary Cooper shows you how to discover and cope with them. Shift your mind into neutral periodically and take regular aerobic exercises to rid yourself of stress and protect or restore your mental powers.

9. How to Boost Your Memory

It is hazardous to mental health—and usually an erroneous diagnosis—to conclude that your memory loss is caused by the onset of senile dementia or Alzheimer's disease. Memory loss can be caused by many factors: low thyroid function and deficiencies of vitamin B–1, B–12, niacin, choline, and the trace minerals, zinc, copper, and boron. It may be difficult to remember where you parked if—in the first place—you didn't take note of the lane number or an object in its line of sight. So when coping with memory problems, review your nutrient intake and use the mnemonic devices offered in this chapter. These devices will help you *and* avoid the embarrassment of forgetting names of people you should remember and other important information.

10. The Answers to Alzheimer's Disease?

Evidence against aluminum in the human system as a cause of Alzheimer's disease is growing. Aluminum assails us in antacids, deodorants, cosmetics, and dozens of other commonly used products. A most threatening source is municipal water which uses alum to settle sediment. Human studies associate aluminum in the brain with symptoms of Alzheimer's disease—neurofibrillary tangles and amyloid. Small amounts of aluminum injected into animal brains brought on all the symptoms of Alzheimer's disease. The fluoride in water and many internally or externally used products can lower the biological availability of acetylcholine by 61 percent. This neurotransmitter is essential to good memory and ability to think clearly.

11. Hormones for the Head

Although every hormone contributes to thinking and remembering, pregnenolone, dehydroepiandrosterone (DHEA), melatonin, and human growth hormone (hGH) are the points of focus in this chapter. Pregnenolone is noted for enhancing memory. Bioneurologist John E. Morley, M.D., of the University of St. Louis, says, "It is, by far, the most potent of the neurosteroids for improving memory by light years."

Although DHEA improves memory, too, it is best known for increasing energy, improving sex life, and contributing to longevity. Melatonin enhances ability to sleep soundly and adjust to jet lag and makes some individuals look and act younger. Therefore, it seems to improve their thinking and memory.

Human growth hormone has an amazing track record for renewing youthfulness, revving up energy and sexual abilities, as well as thinking processes—particularly memory. Edmund Chein, M.D., of the Palm Springs Life Extension Institute, has a phenomenal record—1,000 successful human growth hormone cases with no failures. He offers an unheard of warranty for success: a renewal of your body-mind youthfulness and significant bone growth for osteoporotics, or your money back. Jim Scheer has interviewed Dr. Chein and Bob Jones, one of his prime patients, who is 69 and looks 42.

12. How to Raise Your Child's I.Q.—Part One

Many primitive cultures assure the birth of intelligent, healthy babies by means of a super-nutritious diet for *both* the prospective mother and father long before they plan pregnancy, something a sophisticated and supposedly knowledgeable society such as ours fails to do.

Recent studies indicate that, if the goal is a highly intelligent healthy infant, bottle feeding doesn't measure up. Breast is best—by far. A gynecologist-obstetrician friend offers his diet for male and female fertility and an intelligent infant. It works. Alcohol, cigarettes, and coffee are best omitted from the mother-to-be's diet for many frightening reasons.

13. How to Raise Your Child's I.Q.—Part Two

A million-student study in New York city demonstrates the value of eliminating junk food from school lunches—a 15 percent gain in intelligence levels. A protein-rich breakfast keeps children's and adults' blood sugar levels (energy) high through noon and their thinking processes elevated. Mothers share their secrets of enriching foods that kids like, such as hamburgers and pizza—a realistic approach.

Special ways to make your chidren more creative are supplied by Japan's Dr. Naka-Mats, the most prolific inventor of all times. Parents offer their methods for stimulating their children's creativity. Over a period of years, one youngster with unique ideas parlayed his spending money into a $25 million a year business. This can happen to *your* children—or YOU!

14. The Summing Up

Highlights of previous chapters were presented.

In the pages you've read, we've supplied you with indepth information from worldwide sources on every aspect of raising your I.Q. skyhigh.

May your thinking processes exceed your greatest expectations! There's more information for you in the Appendix that follows. However, at this point, let us say it has been our pleasure to be with you throughout this book.

Best of luck and blessings!

Stephen Langer, M.D., and James F. Scheer

APPENDIX

Exotic Brain Boosters

"Smart drugs" may be the new bright hope for boosting I.Q. and memory. Certain doctors now prescribe them for dealing with senile dementia and Alzheimer's disease—occasionally with encouraging results.

However slowly, their use is also spreading to groups not in desperate brain-degenerative conditions: college students whose grades may make or break their job opportunities; professionals finding it difficult to assimilate the almost overwhelming volume of new information, and executives slipping in their ability to remember and make sound decisions.

Some individuals I know reason that they need smart drugs, because they provide a faster track today, and they want to gain that competitive edge.

Yet to most individuals the mention of smart drugs starts a red flag waving frantically in their minds. Danger! This response is understandable. Smart drugs are often confused with recreational drugs such as marijuana, cocaine, heroin, and speed that give the illusion of boosting the mind and, if used habitually, may actually handicap it or even cause brain damage.

Look at ads for prescription drugs in medical journals. Note the long list of "contraindications"—medical jargon for side effects. All are worth noting. Some drugs bring on horrendous side effects, among them a high blood pressure medicine that makes men impotent, a drug to prevent premature birth that may result in physically or mentally defective babies, or tranquilizers said to drive takers to commit suicide or murder.

From Where I Sit

As a medical doctor who created and launched the first drug-detox program for a northern California county—one used as a model for other counties and states—I can help clarify the possible benefits and hazards of taking smart drugs. I hope my views here will prove helpful.

Some smart drugs have met the challenge. Some haven't. Others are still being evaluated. Here though are five of the drugs that have earned the best reviews from qualified people.

It is important to recall that "smart drugs" do several things: improve blood circulation to the brain, increase metabolism, encourage the growth of the brain cells' mini tree-like branches (dendrites), supply biochemical raw materials for synthesizing brain neurotransmitters, and clean out age pigments (lipofuscin, that accumulates in the brain and forms brown spots on the hands and on the face).

Discovered in the 1950s by Dr. Joseph Knoll, a Hungarian pharmacologist, *deprenyl*—also known as Eldepryl or selegiline—is a chemical relative of amphetamine. It is FDA-approved for managing Parkinson's disease, an ailment characterized by motor dysfunction, tremors, and poor balance.

Parkinson's disease attacks neurotransmitters that produce dopamine and impairs the mind. Dopamine is essential for retaining control of muscle movements and balance. Dopamine loses efficiency due to the normal aging process. Parkinson's disease, however, hurries this deterioration.

Although deprenyl controls and slows the progress of Parkinson's disease, it is not a cure. The most effective therapy for Parkinson's disease is L–dopa to build up the brain's rapidly reduced supply of dopamine.

Deprenyl is a derivative of phenylethylamine (PEA), found in inordinate amounts in brains of people in love. As a result, it is known as the love chemical. It is also an ingredient in chocolate. Whether it be love or lust, old male rats on deprenyl have been revived sexually, as observed by their renewed interest in sex and by mounting frequency.[1]

Deprenyl Boosts Antioxidants

Deprenyl also helps the formation of superoxide dismutase (SOD) and catalase, two powerhouse antioxidants that protect both the neurons that release the neurotransmitter dopamine and dopamine itself. It quenches free radical activities that reduce brain function.[2]

Although various researchers believe deprenyl can manage Alzheimer's disease, few doctors risk prescribing it, because it is not approved by the FDA for Alzheimer's disease and because they fear malpractice suits.

Beverly Potter and Sebastian Orfali in their book *Brain Boosters,* however, tell of the successful treatment of three old dogs afflicted with dementia like that in aged human beings. The dogs wandered around aimlessly, no longer recognized familiar people, and sometimes lost bladder control.[3]

A study by David Bruyette, assistant professor at Kansas State University's College of Veterinary Medicine, revealed that a deprenyl-based, patented drug that he fed them transformed the dogs to normal.

Exotic Brain Boosters 215

In various experiments, deprenyl has also shown indications of extending the life span of human beings. Its discoverer, Dr. Knoll, indicates that deprenyl makes a person more alert, energetic, positive-minded and sexually motivated.

How Deprenyl Works

To understand how deprenyl works and may help Alzheimer's disease patients, it is important to know that there must be a balance of chemicals at work in the human brain. When we are in such a balance, we are mentally alert, have abundant mental and physical energy, remember well, and have the feeling that all's right with the world.

A substance called monamine oxidase (MAO) helps us keep a proper balance of brain chemicals. The amount of MAO rises, however, as we age. In the case of Alzheimer's disease patients, it skyrockets, and quickly "gobbles up" brain chemicals essential to efficient thinking and remembering, to emotional stability, and to the ability to care for oneself.

Deprenyl reduces the action of MAO, so that brain chemicals can again move toward a harmonious balance.

The writers of *Brain Boosters* state that "Alzheimer's sufferers treated with deprenyl demonstrate significant improvements in cognitive behavior and neuroendocrine function with few side effects...."[4]

Although deprenyl helps Alzheimer's patients to concentrate, learn, and remember better, it is not a cure.

Accelerated Sluggish Thinking

Another smart drug that boosts intelligence and charges up the central nervous system is *piracetam*. One of my new patients who had a prescription for piracetam from his previous doctor told me the following:

"My thinking was sluggish. My memory was shot."

A part-time actor who once had a phenomenal memory—dialogue would race through his mind automatically—slowly began to lose it and his confidence.

"I would doze off at my desk after lunch as if I hadn't slept the night before. Then it all changed. The first time I took piracetam I couldn't believe what happened. My mind had a jump start."

An instant response is anything but typical about piracetam. Usually the change is slow and progressively noticeable. Piracetam fills several acute needs for aging brains. With diminished blood flow delivering less oxygen to the brain—or even within a stroke—piracetam guards brain cells against oxygen starvation. This support gives the brain time to recover.[5]

Piracetam speeds up the metabolic rate of the brain and its energy level.[6] A revealing study spotlights what could be a significant ability of piracetam. Fed piracetam for two weeks, old rats developed an increase of 30 to 40 receptors in their frontal cortexes—indicating that the drug is apparently able to regenerate the nervous system.[7]

Piracetam accelerates learning and memory in healthy individuals and also persons with memory deficits.[8] Animal and human studies verify that piracetam speeds up learning and enhances memory. Rats treated with this smart drug quickly learned to avoid areas where they were given a mild electric shock. Untreated rats were slower in avoiding the shock areas.[9]

In an experiment, students taking 4.8 grams of piracetam daily for two weeks showed a "significant improvement" over placebo-takers in remembering verbal information.[10]

Convincing Research

Another study tested 18 middle-aged individuals who were healthy, except for a bad memory. After four weeks on 4.8 grams of piracetam daily, they showed a marked memory improvement.[11]

All studies of this smart brain product show that it is equally effective in enhancing thinking and memory of animals and human beings of all ages.

If your problem is brain fatigue, piracetam may be able to help you. Along with aging, most people experience a lessening of the amount of adenosine triphosphate (ATP) available for conversion into energy. Brain cells depend upon the continuous building up and breaking down of ATP for energy.

When there's too little ATP, enzymes in the cells are hardly able to spark the release of energy. Progressive cardiovascular doctors have found piracetam invaluable for treating stroke victims or others who have sustained brain damage.

Although piracetam may be new to you, it is an old faithful to many biochemists. Various studies performed with it show that it appears to have minimal side effects, if taken as directed. A small minority of people experience gastrointestinal upset, nausea, or sleeplessness. Still, this smart drug is not toxic. It may possibly increase the effects of other drugs—particularly amphetamines, the smart drug hydergine, and some psychotropics.

Piracetam is available in various European countries for ailments such as alcoholism, anemia, dementia, dyslexia, senile dementia, sickle cell anemia, stroke, and vertigo. At this time, it has not been approved by the FDA for use in the United States.

Hydergine's Change of Life

Another brain booster, *Hydergine,* started out its chemical life as a reducer of high blood pressure, particularly in pregnant women. When it was used for patients of advanced years, more happened than the reduction of hypertension.

Oldsters reported the return of a lost memory, increased ability to think more clearly, and improved mood and morale. Researchers took notice. This was more than a blood pressure medicine!

Hydergine can do many things for many brain problems: guarding the brain from harm when the oxygen supply is low; enhancing the brain's ability to use oxygen efficiently; and aiding protein synthesis and nerve growth factor, key functions in brain regeneration.

Earlier we mentioned how stimulating environments—frequently supplied new toys for Dr. Marian Diamond's rats—stimulated the growth of dendrites in brain cells. In numerous experiments, Hydergine has been found to do the same thing. Proliferating dendrites help make better connections between brain cells, sharpening thinking and remembering.

Hydergine super-charges brain energy and performs another valuable service. It eliminates lipofuscin (aging pigments). This biological sludge can block neurotransmitters, reducing or cutting off communication lines. Over and above this, Hydergine is an antioxidant that keeps free radicals from injuring or disabling brain cells.

Long Track Record

One of the most researched smart drugs of all, Hydergine has been studied by the Sandoz Corporation since the 1940s. It is now among the leading treatments for senility and has shown some effectiveness in Alzheimer's disease.[12]

What are effective dosages for Hydergine? In the United States, doctors generally prescribe three milligrams daily. In Europe the usual dosages are nine milligrams in three divided doses. Patients report no marked changes for two to three months. Hydergine's occasional side effects include headache, nausea, and upset stomach. An overdose can produce an effect similar to amnesia. People allergic to it or with an acute chronic psychosis are steered away from it by their doctors.

Although Hydergine is a prescription item in the United States, many doctors are familiar only with its uses for high blood pressure and for senile dementia. Very few prescribe it to patients of any age for the enhancement of thinking and remembering.

Imitation of a Natural Hormone

Like Hydergine, *vasopressin*, called Diapid, another prescription drug, is growing in popularity. It is sometimes called "the memory hormone." Vasopressin is secreted by the pituitary gland.

Research of this smart drug was launched in 1965 by Dr. David de Wied, of the University of Utrecht in the Netherlands. In animal experiments, he discovered that this hormone helps to imprint new information in the brain's memory centers.[13] He discovered that no new information can be acquired without vasopressin's biochemical contributions.

Numerous studies in the past generation have shown striking effects on cognition and memory of vasopressin and have been validated: a substantial improvement in long-term memory; a marked enhancement of ability to pay attention, concentrate, recognize, retain, and recall. It has proved helpful in memory-impaired patients and in normal aging individuals. Vasopressin has been successful in memory enhancement of people with head injuries as well as young and old healthy subjects.

In *Mind Food and Smart Pills*, Ross Pelton, R.Ph., Ph.D., writes the following[14]:

"One study of young, healthy subjects (college volunteers) documented the effects of vasopressin on memory."

The first group of students was given vasopressin, and the other was given a placebo. Those treated with vasopressin demonstrated significant increases in learning ability and memory.

A legitimate stage actor I know took vasopressin for several months before he had to learn his lines for a new play. "It's invaluable when you have lots of new information to memorize," he told me. "I learn my part in a fraction of the time that I took before using vasopressin. I like it very much because it actually is a hormone made by the brain."

As for side effects, those of vasopressin are usually not extreme: abdominal discomfort (sometimes cramps), increased bowel movements, headaches, nasal itching, eye-watering, and a runny nose. Vasopressin should be avoided by pregnant women, hypertensive people, and epileptics.

A typical daily dosage of vasopressin is 12 to 16 USP units or three to four squirts of the spray form in the nasal passage. It is available by prescription. The *Physician's Desk Reference* reports only the conventional usage of this hormone: for coping with the frequent need to urinate in cases of diabetes insipidus and children's bedwetting. These are the two uses approved by the FDA. (Please remember that this chapter is for *information only.*)

Most doctors limit themselves to going by the book and won't stretch a point and write a prescription for anything but its FDA-approved use.

Why Vincamine Is So Widely Used

Among persons familiar with the full range of smart drugs, *vincamine* is one of the most popular, not only because it enhances thinking and remembering, but because it is derived from an herb, periwinkle, and is low-cost.

Again, authors Beverly Potter and Sebastian Orfali show

that vincamine charges up brain metabolism in several ways: increases blood flow, increases the rate at which brain cells produce ATP (the cell molecule that creates energy); and accelerates the brain's use of glucose and oxygen.[15]

They state that Gedeon Richter, a Hungarian company that markets this product, "has funded more than a hundred studies to show its effectiveness and safety." Their research has shown that vincamine is a potent aid for memory improvement. In instances of cerebral insufficiency, patients could remember more words after being treated. At the start, they could recall only six out of ten words on a list. However, after using vincamine, most patients remembered every word on the list.

The usual dosage prescribed was 5 to 10 milligrams daily. Beneficial results are sometimes slow in coming—usually in about a year. Mild stomach upset is the one of few negative factors that is reported relative to vincamine. It is available only by prescription in this country.

Summary

According to my evaluations of smart drugs, the five described in these pages—deprenyl, piracetam, Hydergine, vasopressin, and vincamine—appear to be the most effective for enhancing learning and memory.

WARNING! Consult with a knowledgeable physician before using these smart drugs or antiaging drugs. There is always an element of risk—particularly if you are taking other medicines.

PLEASE NOTE: We do not recommend smart drugs. We have included them for the sake of this book's completeness: for information only.

New information, products, and tests are constantly becoming available. If you wish to receive free information about them from time to time, please send a self-addressed, stamped business size envelope to:

Peak Performance
P.O. Box 1549
Lafayette, CA 94549

References

Chapter 1 Making of a Genius

1. Rivera, Robert, Personal communication.
2. Vercruyssen, Max, "You Learn Better While Standing," News story from the University of Southern California, March 12, 1984.
3. "Rocket Fuel for the Brain," *Exec,* Spring 1995, pp. 55–56.
4. Shay, K.A., "Shoring Up the Aging Mind," *Health and Wellness Top 40 Research Report,* July 1992.
5. Khalsa, Darma Singh, M.D., Press meeting, American Academy for the Advancement of Medicine, Las Vegas, NV, December 13, 1997.
6. Kolata, Gina, "Does Brain Exercise Work?" *New York Times Magazine,* October 6, 1991.
7. "Research on Stress Hormones: Powerful Agents in Health and Disease," Salk Institute Newsletter, 1986, pp. 2–3.
8. Langer, Stephen E., M.D., and Scheer, James F., *Solved: The Riddle of Illness,* Second Edition (New Canaan, CT: Keats Publishing, Inc., 1995), pp. 4–5.

Chapter 2 Exercise the Brain for Better Thinking!

1. Lombard, Jay, M.D., and Germano, Carl, *The Brain Wellness Plan* (New York: Kensington Books, 1997), pp. 11–12.
2. Lal, Gobind Behari, "Brain 'Exercise' Stimulates Growth," Science Service, November 15, 1964.
3. Diamond, Marian, Personal communication, February 1985.
4. Boorsalis, Maria G. et al., "Acute Phase Response and Plasma Carotenoid Concentrations in Elderly Women: Findings from a Nuns' Study," *Applied Nutritional Investigation*, 1996, 12: 475–478.
5. Ceci, Stephen, "Time in School Boosts Intelligence," News story from Cornell University, January 1992.
6. Schaie, Warner, Personal communication, December 1994.

Chapter 3 The Importance of Being Oxygenated

1. Masor, Nathan, M.D., *The New Psychiatry* (New York: Philosophical Library, 1959), pp. 99–100.
2. Williams, Roger J., *Free and Unequal* (Austin, TX: University of Texas Press, 1953), p. 9.
3. ———, *Biochemical Individuality* (New York: John Wiley & Sons, 1956), pp. 30–31.
4. Langer, Stephen E., M.D., and Scheer, James F., *Solved: The Riddle of Illness*, Second Edition (New Canaan, CT: Keats Publishing, Inc., 1995), p. 6.
5. Berman, Louis, M.D., *The Glands Regulating Personality* (New York: The Macmillan Company, 1921), p. 55.
6. Horrobin, David, "Essential Fatty Acids and Aging," Technical Information Bulletin 15: Efamol Series, 1980.
7. Masor, Nathan, M.D., *The New Psychiatry* (New York: Philosophical Library, 1959), pp. 99–100.
8. Langer, Stephen E., M.D., and Scheer, James F., *Solved:*

The Riddle of Illness, Second Edition (New Canaan, CT: Keats Publishing, Inc., 1995), p. 42.
9. Garrison, Jr., Robert A. and Somer, Elizabeth, *The Nutrition Desk Reference,* Third Edition (New Canaan, CT: Keats Publishing, Inc., 1995), pp. 198–199.
10. Donchin, Emanuel and Marshall, Noel K., "A Chilling Effect," *Psychology Today,* February 1982, p. 92.
11. U.S. Department of Agriculture, "Conquest of Pernicious Anemia," *Food: The Yearbook of Agriculture,* (Washington, D.C.: Government Printing Office, 1959), p. 163.

Chapter 4 Nutrients That Skyrocket Your I.Q.

1. Cheraskin, E., Ringsdorf, W.M. and Clark, J.W., *Diet and Disease* (New Canaan, CT: Keats Publishing, Inc., 1968), pp. 177–178.
2. Rodale, J.I., "Vitamin B-1 and Mentality Go Together," *Prevention Magazine,* March 1970, p. 38.
3. Bell, Elizabeth C., Ph.D., "Prevention: The Relation of Nutrition to Mental Health," *Journal of Psychology,* April 1958, Vol. 45, 1061, pp. 47–74.
4. Spies, T.C., "Some Recent Advances in Nutrition," *Journal of the American Medical Association,* June 7, 1958, 167: 6, pp. 675–690.
5. Rodale, J.I., *The Complete Book of Nutrition* (Emmaus, PA: Rodale Books, Inc., 1961), pp. 760–763.
6. Elwood, Catharyn, *Feel Like a Million* (Old Greenwich, CT: Devin Adair, 1956), pp. 234–235.
7. Ibid., p. 258.
8. Rogers, Lorene, Ph.D., and Pelton, Ross B., "Effect of Glutamine on I.Q. Scores of Mentally Deficient Children," Texas Reports on Biology and Medicine, 1957, Vol. 15, No. 1, pp. 84–90.
9. McFarland, Judy Lindbergh, *Aging Without Growing*

Old (Palos Verdes, CA: Western Front Publishing, 1997), p. 141.
10. Wurtman, R.J., "Nutrients That Modify Brain Function," *Scientific American*, 1982 246(4), pp. 50–59.
11. Pines, Maya, "What You Eat Can Affect Your Brain," *Reader's Digest*, September 1993, pp. 54–58.
12. Liang, Pek Hien et al., "Undernutrition in Infancy and Childhood Limits Mentality," *American Journal of Clinical Nutrition*, December 1967.
13. Golub, M.S. et al., "Developmental Zinc Deficiency and Behavior," *Journal of Nutrition*, 1995, 125: 2263S–2271S.
14. "Zinc Deficiency Affects The Memory," News story issued by the University of Texas Medical Branch at Galveston, March 1991.
15. Editors of *Prevention, Future Youth* (Emmaus, PA: Rodale Press, 1987), pp. 265–266.
16. Root, Elizabeth and Longenecker, John, Personal communication, November 1997.
17. Cranton, E. M. and Frackelton, J.P., "Treatment of Free Radical Pathology in Chronic Degenerative Disease with EDTA Chelation," *Journal of Holistic Medicine*, 1984.
18. Pelton, Ross, Ph.D., *Mind Food and Smart Pills* (San Diego: T & R Press, 1986), p. 33.

Chapter 5 Brain Transplant or Something Better?

1. Atkins, Robert C., *Dr. Atkins' Vita-Nutrient Solution* (New York: Simon & Schuster, 1998), p. 253.
2. Crook, T.H. et al., "Effects of Phosphatidylserine on Age-Associated Memory Impairment," *Neurology*, 1991, 41: 644–49.
3. Huguet, F. et al., "Decreased Cerebral 5–HT 1A Receptors During Aging: Reversal by Ginkgo Biloba Ex-

tract," *Journal of Pharmacy and Pharmacology,* 1994, 46: 316–18.
4. Murphree, H.B. et al., "The Stimulating Effect of 2 Dimethylaminoethanol (Deanol) in Human Volunteer Subjects,' *Clinical Pharmacology and Therapeutics,* 1960, Vol. 1, pp. 303–310.
5. Pfeiffer, Carl C., M.D., et al., "Stimulant Effect of 2–Dimethyl–Aminoethanol: Possible Precursor of Brain Acetylcholine," *Science* 126 (1957): 610–611.
6. Dean, Ward, M.D., Morgenthaler, John and Fowkes, Stephen, *Smart Drugs: The Next Generation* (Menlo Park, CA: Health Freedom Publications, 1990), p. 36.
7. Ibid.
8. Passwater, Richard, Ph.D., *Evening Primrose Oil* (New Canaan, CT: Keats Publishing, Inc., 1980), p. 12.

Chapter 6 CATS and Your Mind

1. Braly, James, M.D., *Dr. Braly's Food Allergy & Nutrition Revolution* (New Canaan, CT: Keats Publishing, Inc., 1992), pp. 240–242.
2. Newbold, H.L., M.D., *Dr. Newbold's Nutrition for Your Nerves* (New Canaan, CT: Keats Publishing, Inc., 1993), p. 138.
3. "No Coffee Regimen Cuts Blood Pressure," *Medical Tribune News Service,* March 8, 1991.
4. "Heavy Drinking and High Stroke Risk," *Science News,* November 1986, p. 276.
5. Ibid.
6. "Alcohol Effects Linked to Body Temperature," News story, University of Southern California, May 12, 1986.
7. Hendler, Sheldon Saul, M.D., Ph.D., *Purification Prescription* (New York: William Morrow & Company, 1991), pp. 36–37.
8. Kershbaum, A. et al., "Effect of Smoking and Nicotine

on Adrenocortical Secretion," *Journal of the American Medical Association,* 1968, 203: 113–116.
9. Pelletier, O., "Smoking and Vitamin C Levels in Humans," *American Journal of Clinical Nutrition,* 1968, 21, pp. 1254–1258.
10. Taub, Harold J., "Better Protection for Smokers' Lungs," *Let's Live,* March 1976, p. 8.
11. Owens, Karen, "Beware of Second-Hand Smoke," News story from K.A. Owens and Associates, October 1987.
12. Ahrens, Richard A., "Sugar and Hypertension," *Journal of Nutrition,* April 1980, pp. 128–131.
13. Stephen Gyland, M.D., Personal communication, March 1983.

Chapter 7 Heavy Metals and Your Brain

1. Raloff, Janet, "Lead May Foster Immune Attack on Brain," *Science News,* January 14, 1995, p. 23.
2. Bower, Bruce, "Excess Lead Linked to Boy's Delinquency," *Science News,* February 10, 1996.
3. Faelton, Sharon, *The Complete Book of Minerals for Health* (Emmaus, PA: Rodale Press, 1981), pp. 175–176.
4. Casdorph, Richard, M.D., and Walker, Morton, M.D., *Toxic Metal Syndrome* (Garden City Park, NY: Avery Publishing Group, 1995), pp. 189–190.
5. Marlowe, Mike, Chairman, Department of Languages, Appalachian State University, Personal communication, January 1998.
6. Murray, Frank, *The Big Family Guide to All the Minerals* (New Canaan, CT: Keats Publishing, Inc., 1995), p. 411.
7. Langer, Stephen E., M.D., and Scheer, James F., *How to Win at Weight Loss* (Rochester, VT: Thorsons Publishers, 1987), p. 81.

Chapter 8 Stress: The Mind-Killer

1. Fackelmann, K.A., "Stress Puts Squeeze on Clogged Vessels," *Science News,* November 16, 1991, p. 309.
2. Bricklin, Mark, *Practical Encyclopedia of Natural Healing* (Emmaus, PA: Rodale Press, 1976), p. 196.
3. Riccitelli, M.L., "Vitamin C Therapy in Geriatric Practice," *Journal of the American Geriatric Society,* January 1972, pp. 49–55.
4. Rath, Matthias and Pauling, Linus, "Solution to the Puzzle of Human Cardiovascular Disease," *Journal of Orthomolecular Medicine,* 1991, 6:125–134.
5. Rath, Matthias and Pauling, Linus, "How to Prevent Heart Attack and Stroke," Linus Pauling Heart Institute, 1992.
6. Cooper Cary, Ph.D., Personal communication.
7. Gerras, Charles (ed.), *The Complete Book of Vitamins* (Emmaus, PA: Rodale Press, 1977), pp. 117–118.
8. Justice, Blair, Ph.D., *Who Gets Sick* (Houston: Peak Press, 1987), pp. 58–60.
9. Gillette, Paul and Hornbeck, Marie, *Psychochemistry* (New York: Warner Paperback, 1974), pp. 96–97.

Chapter 9 How to Boost Your Memory

1. Wentzler, Rick, *The Vitamin Book* (New York: Gramercy Publishing Company, 1978), p. 43.
2. Gerras, Charles (ed.), *The Complete Book of Vitamins* (Emmaus, PA: Rodale Press, Inc.), pp. 162–164.
3. Adelle Davis, Personal communication.
4. Holmes, A.J., McDonald, "Dietary Deficiency of Vitamin B–12 in Relation to Mental and Emotional Symptoms," *British Medical Journal,* Vol. 5006, pp. 1395–1398.
5. Lindenbaum, John et al., "Neuropsychiatric Disorders Caused by Cobalamin Deficiency in the Absence of

Anemia or Macrocytosis," *New England Journal of Medicine,* June 30, 1988: 318 (26): 1720–1728.

6. Jennings, Isobel, *Vitamins in Endocrine Metabolism* (Springfield, IL: Charles C. Thomas Publishers, 1970), pp. 41–46.

7. "Vitamin B–12 Supplements Better Absorbed than Same Vitamin In Foods," News story, University of Southern California, January 1987.

8. Bartus, R.T., M.D., et al., "Memory Deficits in Aged Cebus Monkeys and Facilitation with Central Cholinomimetics," *Neurobiology of Aging,* 1980, 1: 145.

9. Bartus, R.T., M.D. et al., "Age-Related Changes on Passive-Avoidance Retention," *Science,* 1980, 209: 301.

10. Passwater, Richard, Ph.D., *The New Supernutrition* (New Canaan, CT: Keats Publishing, Inc., 1993), pp. 55–56.

11. Hochschild, R., "Effect of Dimethylaminoethanol on Life Span of Senile Male A/J Mice," *Experimental Geriatrics,* 1973, Vol. 6, pp. 185–191.

12. Pelton, Ross, *Mind Food and Smart Pills* (San Diego, CA: T & R, 1986), p. 67.

13. Murphree, H.B. et al., "The Stimulant Effect of 2–Dimethylaminoethanol (Deanol) in Human Volunteer Subjects," *Clinical Pharmacy and Therapeutics* 1, 1960: 303–310.

14. Potter, Beverly and Orfali, Sebastian, *Brain Boosters* (Berkeley, CA: Ronin Publishing, Inc., 1993), p. 118.

15. Cipolli, C. and Chiari, G., "Effects of L–acetylcholine on Mental Deterioration in the Aged," *Clinica Terapeutica* 132: 479–510.

16. Lino, A. et al., "Psycho-Functional Changes in Attention and Learning Under the Action of L–acetyl–carnitine in 17 Young Subjects," *Clinica Terapeutica* 140: 569–73.

17. Grioli, S. et al., "Pyroglutamic Acid Improves the Age Associated Memory Impairment," *Fundamental Clinical Pharmacology* 4: 169–73.
18. Justice, Blair, *Who Gets Sick* (Houston: Peak Press, 1987), p. 89.
19. McBride, Judy, "Diets Deficient in Boron Can Dull the Senses," USDA News Feature, April 19, 1990.
20. "Zinc-Iron Supplements Boost Memory," News story, University of Texas Medical Branch at Galveston, July 1991.

Chapter 10 The Answers to Alzheimer's Disease?

1. Pfeiffer, Carl C., *Mental and Elemental Nutrients* (New Canaan, CT: Keats Publishing, Inc., 1975), p. 308.
2. McLaughlan, D.R. et al., "Alterations in Short-Term Retention, Conditioned Avoidance Response Acquisition and Motivation Following Aluminum-Induced Neurofibrillary Degeneration," *Physiology and Behavior,* 1973, 10: 925–933.
3. Salaman, Maureen and Scheer, James F., *Foods That Heal* (Menlo Park, CA: Statford Publishing, 1989), p. 30.
4. Alfrey, Allen C., et al., "The Dialysis Encephalopathy Syndrome: Possible Aluminum Intoxication," *New England Journal of Medicine,* January 22, 1976: 185–86.
5. Murray, Frank, *The Big Family Guide to All the Minerals* (New Canaan, CT: Keats Publishing, Inc., 1995), p. 376.
6. Murray, Richard P., "Does Aluminum Toxicity Contribute to Alzheimer's Disease?" *Health Freedom News,* February 1994, p. 13.
7. Casdorph, H. Richard, M.D., and Walker, Morton, *Toxic Metal Syndrome* (Garden City Park, NY: Avery Publishing Group, 1995), p. 85.

8. Johnson, Robert J., "Aluminum: A Threat to Mental Health," *Bestways,* December 1986, p. 28.
9. Raloff, Janet, "New Alzheimer's Theory," *Science News,* April 18, 1981, p. 45.
10. ———, September 15, 1984, p. 167.
11. Casdorph, H. Richard, M.D., and Walker, Morton, *Toxic Metal Syndrome* (Garden City Park, NY: Avery Publishing Group, 1995), pp. 10–13.
12. Justice, Blair, *Who Gets Sick* (Houston: Peak Press, 1987), p. 11.
13. Wurtman, R.J., "Nutrients That Modify Brain Function," *Scientific American,* 246 (4) pp. 50–59.
14. Raloff, Janet, "Behavioral Improvement of Alzheimer's Patients," *Science News,* July 13, 1985, p. 24.
15. Ibid.
16. Morgan, Brian L.G., M.D., *Nutrition Prescription* (New York: Crown Publishers, 1988), p. 27.
17. Zeavin, Edna, "Foods That Influence Human Behavior," *Bestways,* September 1985, p. 11.
18. Boorsalis, Maria G. et al., "Acute Phase Response and Plasma Carotene Concentration in Elderly Women: Findings from a Nuns' Study," *Applied Nutritional Investigation,* 1996, 12: 475–476.

Chapter 11 Hormones for the Head

1. Regelson, William, M.D., and Colman, Carol, *The Super-Hormone Promise* (New York: Pocket Books, 1996), p. 72.
2. Sahelian, Ray, *Pregnenolone* (Garden City Park, NY: Avery Publishing Group, 1997), p. 41.
3. Regelson, William, M.D., and Colman, Carol, *The Super-Hormone Promise* (New York: Pocket Books, 1996), p. 74.
4. Ibid.
5. Flood, J.F. et al., "Memory-Enhancing Effects in Male

Mice of Pregnenolone and Steroids Metabolically Derived From It," *Proceedings of the National Academy of Science,* 1992, 89: 1567–1571.

6. Flood, J.F. et al., "Pregnenolone Sulfate Enhances Post-Training Memory Processes When Injected in Low Doses Into Limbic System Structures," *Proceedings of the National Academy of Science,* 1995, 92:10806–10818.

7. Roberts, Eugene, "Pregnenolone: From Selye to Alzheimer and a Model of the Pregnenolone Sulfate-Binding Site on the GABA Receptor," *Biochemical Pharmacology,* 1995, 49: 1–16.

8. Sahelian, Ray, *Pregnenolone* (Garden City Park, NY: Avery Publishing Group, 1998), P. 23.

9. Klatz, Ronald, Talk at Annual Meeting of the American Academy of Anti-Aging Medicine, Las Vegas, NV, December 12–14, 1997.

10. Ibid.

11. Klatz, Ronald, *Grow Young With hGH* (New York: HarperCollins Publishers, 1997), p. 146.

12. Ibid., pp. 73–74.

13. Ibid., p. 141.

14. Deijen, J.B. et al., "Cognitive Impairment and Mood Disturbance in Growth Hormone Deficiency in Men," in preparation, December 1997.

15. Rudman, D. et al., "Effects of Human Growth Hormone in Men Over 60 Years Old," *New England Journal of Medicine,* July 5, 1990, 323: 1–6.

16. Ibid.

17. Rudman, D. et al., "Effects of Human Growth Hormone on Body Composition in Elderly Men," *Hormone Research,* 1991, 36 suppl 1: 73–81.

Chapter 12 How to Raise Your Child's I.Q.—Part One

1. Price, Weston, D.D.S., *Nutrition and Physical Degeneration* (Los Angeles: American Academy of Applied Nutrition, 1945), p. 401–402.
2. Ibid., pp. 397–403.
3. "Mother's Milk Boosts I.Q.s of Babies," *Townsend Letter for Doctors,* August/September 1996, p. 11.
4. Raloff, Janet, "Women and Alcohol: A Gastric Disadvantage," *Science News,* January 20, 1990, p. 39.
5. Williams, Roger J., *Nutrition Against Disease* (New York: Bantam Books, 1982), p. 178.

Chapter 13 How to Raise Your Child's I.Q.—Part Two

1. "Vitamin-IQ Link Has Parents Pushing Pills," *San Francisco Chronicle,* October 10, 1988, Sec. 5, p. 5.
2. Schoenthaler, Stephen, Ph.D., Doraz, Walter and Wakefield, James, Jr., "Impact of Low Food Additives and Sucrose Diets on Academic Performance in 803 New York City Public Schools," *International Journal of Biosocial Research,* v. 8, no. 2, 1986, pp. 185–195.
3. Albrecht, William A., "Diseases vs. Deficiencies via the Soil," *Natural Food and Farming Digest,* 1957, pp. 106–109.
4. Braly, James, M.D., *Dr. Braly's Food Allergy and Diet Revolution* (New Canaan, Ct.: Keats Publishing, Inc., 1992), p. 47.
5. Monmaney, Terence, "Medications Kill 100,000 Annually, Study Says," *Los Angeles Times,* April 15, 1998.
6. Kahan, Barbara, *Healthier Children* (New Canaan, Ct.: Keats Publishing, Inc., 1990), p. 157.
7. Orent-Keiles, E. and Hallman, L.F., "The Breakfast Meal in Relation to Blood Sugar Values," U.S. Department of Agriculture, Circular 827.
8. "Reverse Heaviest Meal for Weight Loss," *Journal*

of the Louisiana State Medical Society, 1985: 137 (6) 35–38.

9. Thompson, Charles "Chick," *What A Great Idea!* (New York: Harper Perennial, 1992), Foreword.

Appendix: Exotic Brain Boosters

1. Potter, Beverly and Orfali, Sebastian, *Brain Boosters* (Berkeley, CA: Ronin Publishing, Inc., 1993), p. 114.
2. Ibid.
3. Ibid., p. 115
4. Ibid., p. 116.
5. Richardson, Alan E., "Effect of Piracetam on Level of Consciousness After Neurosurgery," *The Lancet*, 1977: 1110–1111.
6. Stegink, A.J., "The Clinical Use of Piracetam, A New Nootropic Drug," Arxneim-Forsch, *Drug Research* 21, no. 6 (1972): 975–77.
7. Dean, Ward, M.D., and Morgenthaler, John, *Smart Drugs and Nutrients* (Santa Cruz, CA: B&J Publications, 1990), p. 40.
8. Dimond, S.J. and Brouwer, E.Y.M., "Increase in the Power of Human Memory in Normal Men Through the Use of Drugs," *Psychopharmacology* 49 (1976): 307–309.
9. Giurgia, C.E. et al., "The Nootropic Approach to the Pharmacology of the Integrative Activity of the Brain," *Conditioned Reflex* (1973) 8, no. 2, 108–115.
10. Dimond, S.J. and Brouwer, E.Y.M., "Increase in the Power of Human Memory in Normal Men Through the Use of Drugs," *Psychopharmaceuticals* 49 (1976) 301–306.
11. Mindus, P. et al., "Piracetam-Induced Improvement in Mental Performance: A Controlled Study on Normally Aging Individuals," ACTA *Psychiatrica Scandinavia* (1976) 54: 150–160.

12. Dean, Ward, M.D., and Morgenthaler, John, *Smart Drugs and Nutrients* (Santa Cruz, CA: B&J Publications, 1990), p. 140.
13. de Wied, D. et al., "Vasopressin and Memory Consolidation," *Perspectives in Brain Research* (New York: Elsevier Scientific Publishing Company, 1975).
14. Pelton, Ross, Ph.D., *Mind Food and Smart Pills* (San Diego: T & R Publishers, 1986), p. 97.
15. Potter, Beverly and Orfali, Sebastian, *Brain Boosters* (Berkeley, CA: Ronin Publishing, Inc., 1993), p. 110.

Recommended Reading

Age Reversal. Edmund Chein. Palm Springs Life Extension Institute. Palm Springs, CA, 1997.

Aging Without Growing Old. Judy Lindbergh McFarland (with Laura McFarland Luczak). Western Front, Palos Verde, CA 1997.

The Big Family Guide to All the Minerals. Frank Murray. Keats Publishing, Inc. New Canaan, CT, 1995.

Biochemical Individuality. Roger J. Williams. John Wiley & Sons. New York, 1956.

Brain Boosters. Beverly Potter and Sebastian Orfali. Ronin Publishing. Berkeley, CA, 1993.

The Brain Wellness Plan. Jay L. Lombard and Carl Germano. Kensington Books. New York, 1997.

The Complete Book of Minerals for Health. Sharon Faelton. Rodale Press. Emmaus, PA, 1981.

DHEA: Fountain of Youth. Beth Ley, BL Publications. Newport Beach, CA, 1996.

Diet and Disease. E. Cheraskin, W.M. Ringsdorf and J.W. Clark. Keats Publishing, Inc. New Canaan, CT, 1968.

Recommended Reading

Dr. Atkins' Vita-Nutrient Solution. Robert C. Atkins. Simon & Schuster. New York, 1998.

Dr. Braly's Food Allergy and Diet Revolution. James Braly. Keats Publishing, Inc. New Canaan, CT, 1992.

Dr. Newbold's Nutrition for Your Nerves. H.L. Newbold. Keats Publishing. New Canaan, CT, 1993.

Eat Smart, Think Smart. Robert Haas. HarperCollins. New York, 1994.

Free and Unequal. Roger J. Williams. University of Texas Press. Austin, TX, 1953.

Food—Your Miracle Medicine. Jean Carper. Harper Perennial. New York, 1993.

Foods That Heal. Maureen Salaman and James F. Scheer. Stratford Publishing. Menlo Park, CA, 1989.

Future Youth. Editors of *Prevention Magazine.* Rodale Press. Emmaus, PA, 1987.

Grow Young With hGH. Ronald Klatz. HarperCollins. New York, 1997.

Healthier Children. Barbara Kahan. Keats Publishing, Inc. New Canaan, CT, 1990.

Mind Food and Smart Pills. Ross Pelton. T&R Press. San Diego, CA, 1986.

The New Psychiatry. Nathan Masor. Philosophical Library. New York, 1959.

The New Supernutrition. Richard Passwater. Keats Publishing, Inc. New Canaan, CT, 1993.

Nutrition Against Disease. Roger J. Williams. Bantam Books. New York, 1982.

Recommended Reading

The Nutrition Desk Reference. Robert Garrison, Jr. and Elizabeth Somer. Keats Publishing, Inc. New Canaan, CT, 1997.

Nutrition Prescription. Brian L.G. Morgan. Crown Publishers. New York, 1988.

Nutrition and Physical Degeneration (6th edition). Weston A. Price. Keats Publishing, Inc. New Canaan, CT, 1997.

The Nutrition Superbook: The Good Fats And Oils (edited by Jean Barilla). Keats Publishing, Inc. New Canaan, CT, 1996.

Pregnenolone (Nature's Feel Good Hormone). Ray Sahelian. Avery Publishing Group. Garden City Park, NY, 1997.

Purification Prescription. Sheldon Saul Hendler. William Morrow & Company. New York, 1991.

Smart Drugs and Nutrients. Ward Dean and John Morgenthaler. B&J Publications. Santa Cruz, CA, 1990.

Smart Drugs: The Next Generation. Ward Dean, John Morgenthaler and Stephen Fowkes. Health Freedom Publications. Menlo Park, CA, 1990.

Smart Nutrients. Abram Hoffer and Morton Walker. Avery Publishing Group. Garden City Park, NY, 1994.

Solved: The Riddle of Illness (Second Edition). Stephen Langer and James F. Scheer. Keats Publishing, Inc. New Canaan, CT, 1995.

The Super-Hormone Promise. William Regelson and Carol Colman. Pocket Books. New York, 1996.

Toxic Metal Syndrome. Richard Casdorph and Morton Walker. Avery Publishing Group. Garden City Park, NY, 1995.

What A Great Idea! Charles "Chick" Thompson. Harper Perennial. New York, 1992.

Who Gets Sick. Blair Justice. Peak Press. Houston, TX, 1987.

ABOUT THE AUTHORS

Steven Langer, M.D., practices Preventive Medicine and Clinical Nutrition in Berkley, California. President and Founder of the American Nutritional Medical Association, a research organization, Dr. Langer is an authority on the thyroid gland and a speaker at national and international medical conferences. He has hosted TV (Family Channel) and radio health/nutrition talk shows and, with James F. Scheer, wrote the perennial best seller *Solved: The Riddle of Illness*. Dr. Langer can be reached for personal consultation at (510) 548-7384.

James F. Scheer has edited three nutrition/health magazines—*Let's Live, Food-Wise* and *Health Freedom News*—and he has written or coauthored 21 published books, among them the million-seller *Foods That Heal* (with Maureen Salaman) and the perennial bestseller *Solved: The Riddle of Illness* (with Stephen Langer, M.D.) One of his books served as the basis for the 60-minute film documentary *The Race for Space*, a nominee for an Academy Award.